Surgery

MW01242535

Umut Sarpel

Surgery

An Introductory Guide

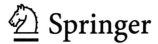 Springer

Umut Sarpel
Department of Surgery
Division of Surgical Oncology
Icahn School of Medicine at Mount Sinai
New York, NY, USA

ISBN 978-1-4939-0902-5   ISBN 978-1-4939-0903-2 (eBook)
DOI 10.1007/978-1-4939-0903-2
Springer New York Heidelberg Dordrecht London

Library of Congress Control Number: 2014940052

Springer is part of Springer Science+Business Media (www.springer.com)

Foreword

Simple can be harder than complex: You have to work hard to get your thinking clean to make it simple. But it's worth it in the end because once you get there, you can move mountains.

— Steve Jobs

Reading this book is like being "scrubbed in" an operation at the elbow of an expert surgeon. This surgeon loves her work. And she has high expectations of you, but she doesn't leave it at that. She is aware of what you have learned so far and what you have not yet encountered. She guides your thinking to enable you to grow into the excellent clinician you aspire to be. Since most students who complete a surgery clerkship will not go on to practice surgery, this may be your only immersion into how to think like a surgeon. Pay attention. This is important.

Dr. Umut Sarpel introduces and demystifies the rhythms and routines of a busy surgical suite, including OR schedules, protocols, and personnel, guiding students to understand the jargon, where and why to focus their attention, how to respond to questions, and quite literally what to do with their hands. Like a good travel guide to an exotic land she translates the colloquial idioms, making the new arrival feel familiar and "semantically competent." This comfort and guidance is critical to learning.

Without guidance a medical student may not figure out what or how to learn in the operating room. Most surgeons highly value the apprenticeship model in the OR, in which trainees learn by doing real-world work alongside an expert. But this model has limits in practice because the master practitioner often fails to speak aloud the hard-earned tacit knowledge critical to understanding the operation. This makes what they do seem mysterious or magical to the novice medical student who is often struck dumb by the foreignness, complexity, and emotional intensity of what is going on. The educational limits of a classic apprenticeship are exacerbated when students, hoping to mimic their teachers, prepare for the OR with what is referred to as "foreground information" rather than ensure that they have mastered the basic background knowledge. This is most noticeable when the student comes to the bedside or operating room having read the latest published literature on surgical technique but can't articulate the indications for the surgery in this patient, the pathophysiology of the disease process, or how to prevent or prepare for the most likely surgical complications.

Skipping the basics can have significant consequences. This is because, as cognitive psychologists have elucidated, the accuracy of clinical decision-making is predicated on the learning of mental models called schemas or scripts. These scripts are foundational structures or patterns of information that are initialized through learning the basics and then become more sophisticated with deliberate practice. Scripts enable the seasoned clinician to instantly and accurately recognize key clinical situations, even when subtle or atypical. Experts have highly detailed and rich scripts, novices very sparse and spotty ones. Without developmentally appropriate scaffolding provided by teachers to ensure these basic scripts are laid down solidly, learning is slowed and some novices may never develop accurate clinical decision-making capacity for the most common surgical diseases.

In this eloquently efficient book, Dr. Umut Sarpel has done the difficult work of simplifying the complex. Ideal instructional materials use text and pictures, are engaging to read, and are aimed just above the current knowledge level of the intended reader—not too low or too high. Sarpel's book does just this. She frames the material in words, images, classic cases, and bulleted lists to help the clinical clerk prepare to learn in the operating room. But this book is not just for students. I believe all surgical educators, especially newly minted ones, need to take a page from this playbook. In fact it would make a great text for faculty development, preparing surgical educators to teach novices about a particular surgical procedure. In addition, all health care professional students such as nurses, physician assistants, and technicians will learn a great deal from this book, which simplifies and explains the most challenging of learning environments.

Umut Sarpel and I have been colleagues and friends for many years. Over that time, I have known her to be a skillful and compassionate physician, wise scholar, and enthusiastic educational leader, but until now I did not have the privilege of knowing her as a teacher. Reading this book, as a General Internist who hasn't been in the OR (except on the table) since I was a clinical clerk in 1982, I have been reminded once again of how challenging it is to learn medicine in complex clinical environments. My respect has redoubled for her compassion and empathy for our students who face a learning challenge akin to drinking from a fire hose. With so many competing demands on their limited time and cognitive energies, many students falter and waste precious time. This book serves as a drinking cup. In the best tradition of academic surgeons, Umut identified an unmet need and then meticulously created this resource. Our students and our patients are better off as a result.

New York, NY   Adina Kalet, M.D., M.P.H.
                                                                   Arnold P. Gold
                            Professor of Humanism and Professionalism
                        Director of the Research on Medical Education
                                                             and Outcomes Unit
            Program on Medical Education Innovation and Research
                              New York University School of Medicine

Preface

A surgical mentor of mine used to advise his medical students "Don't act like tourists!" He wanted them to get deeply immersed in their surgical clerkship, to view themselves as vital members of the surgical team, rather than be passive observers who simply watched surgeons work. Of course, this is easier said than done. The tempo of a surgical service is fast and the rotation is already over by the time you figure out how everything runs.

The operating room—the heart of a medical student's surgical experience—is perhaps the most inscrutable and intimidating aspect of the entire rotation. You will be assigned to cases and will be expected to "read-up" on the operation before scrubbing in. Although this sounds like a simple instruction, in my experience, most students do not really understand how to prepare for a case. Often a student will arrive to my OR having read the latest phase III clinical trial on the disease, but with little knowledge about the patient or understanding of the operation at hand. Participating in an operation has the potential to be one of the most profound learning experiences in all of medical school, but often seems to pass by in a blur.

So, how can you get the most out of your time in the OR? What does it mean to "read-up" on a case? It means that you should know the patient's story, be prepared to discuss the pathophysiology of the disease, understand why this procedure is being performed, be familiar with the main steps of the case, recognize the key anatomy, and be aware of the most common complications of the operation. This task requires you to pull together information from several different sources: texts on anatomy and pathology, surgical atlases, and clinical guidebooks. But even this type of diligent preparation does not take into account last-minute changes in the OR schedule. Surgery is a fast-paced field and it is not unusual to be suddenly reassigned to a new operation or to have an emergency case arise.

The concept of this book was to bring together those various pieces of information that a medical student needs to critically understand an operation, and present it in a unified, concise, efficient, and portable format. Throughout the book, the emphasis is on the use of keywords, diagrams, and illustrations in order to enhance your ability to quickly absorb and retain the relevant information. Each chapter consists of several sections, including:

Introduction: Just-enough information is presented on each of the common indications for an operation and the relevant pathophysiology. The emphasis is on clinical knowledge over basic science facts, and the aspects that are important to surgical decision-making are stressed. Keywords are placed in bold throughout the text, allowing you to quickly find the information you need.

Surgical Technique: Most surgical manuals target the surgical resident, providing technical information that is far too detailed for the needs of a medical student. Nevertheless, some knowledge of the steps of an operation is important for a student to understand the progression of a procedure. In this work, the main steps of each operation are listed, allowing you to follow the case, and interact with your surgical team.

Complications: Perhaps the most important aspect of an operation is what might happen after the skin has been closed. What are the most common complications and how do they present? Despite its significance, this information is rarely covered in medical school texts.

Classic Case: Each chapter ends with a classic case, since a patient story often sticks in the memory longer than does didactic text. These scenarios describe how a patient's symptoms presented, how the disease was diagnosed, and whether complications occurred after surgery.

OR Questions: "Pimping" the student during a case is one of the traditions of surgery. Each chapter in this book ends with several questions that draw your attention to key concepts or often-asked questions.

Anatomy: In traditional anatomy atlases, every anatomical structure in a region is exhaustively listed, whereas only a few of these vessels or nerves may be relevant to a particular operation. In this manual, a color illustration of the operative field accompanies each chapter, and only the structures germane to the operation are identified and labeled. These diagrams have been drawn from the vantage point of the surgeon, rather than an anatomist. In other words, the gallbladder and its blood supply are depicted the way they appear during laparoscopic cholecystectomy, rather than during a cadaveric dissection. This orientation will allow you to recognize the structures that you have learned and follow the course of the operation.

Radiologic Correlation: The ability to read cross-sectional imaging such as CT scans is often not formally taught in the preclinical years, but is an integral part of a surgical rotation. Each chapter in this book provides a typical image of the disease process, allowing you to recognize similarities to your own patient's imaging.

Summary: Finally, each chapter ends with a brief bulleted list that provides a visual, concise summary of the information described in the text. Also included is a list of what perioperative orders are appropriate for the type of surgery. These lists serve as a useful review of the concepts described in the text, and also allow quick access to the vital information if you only have a short time to prepare before your case.

A caveat — this book is certainly not sufficient to carry you through your rotation unsupplemented. It is not intended to be the definitive source for your surgical fund of knowledge; in many cases factual detail has been intentionally sacrificed in order to allow for easier comprehension. The purpose of this work is to bring together the information necessary for you to be an active participant in the operating theater. The better prepared you are for an operation, the more you will get out of the experience.

New York, NY   Umut Sarpel, M.D., M.Sc.

Acknowledgments

This book came to be through the generous help of many people along the way. First of all, I must thank Dr. Zeynel A. Karcıoğlu who resurrected this work from a stalled project by insisting that I show it to his editor at Springer. Without his encouragement, this book would certainly have never seen the light of day. And thank you to that editor, Richard A. Hruska, who took on the project of a neophyte, and stuck with me despite numerous lapsed deadlines. I would like to acknowledge Michael D. Sova, my developmental editor, who suffered through the quotidian emails, questions, and excuses about said deadlines. I must also thank the art department at Springer for transforming my rough sketches into such clear anatomical illustrations.

I am deeply grateful to Dr. Adina Kalet for her offer to write the forward for this book, and for her friendship and mentorship over the years. As a nationally recognized expert in medical education, I particularly appreciate her validation of this project. I also thank Dr. Ageliki Vouyouka, who graciously reviewed the sections on vascular surgery.

Whatever I have learned about surgery over the years, I learned inside the walls of The Mount Sinai Hospital and Bellevue Hospital in New York City. I would like to thank the staff and nurses at these two institutions and especially the patients whose stories and radiologic images populate this book. It also goes without saying that I owe a tremendous amount to all the surgeons who trained me during my residency and fellowship, and who mentored me during my years as a junior attending. Teaching often goes both ways; indeed I have learned just as much from my students and residents over the years. There are simply too many people to name individually.

Thank you to the staff at Vineapple in Brooklyn, who provided me a quiet place to work and plied me with the caffeine to help me accomplish the task.

I must thank my parents, of course for their support and encouragement, but even more so for their eagle-eyed proof reading and suggestions for improvement. Also thank you to my brother Dr. Dost Sarpel for his free advice on all things involving Infectious Diseases.

Finally, I am indebted to my husband, Dr. Ozan Aksoy, who worked alongside me through much of the process, always keeping me on task. And who—despite being the "other kind of doctor"—read through each and every chapter to help me meet my final deadline. Thank you.

Contents

1

Preparing for the OR

Being allowed to participate in an operation comes with the responsibility of learning everything about your patient's medical history. In exchange for scrubbing into cases, you will be expected to know the story of how your patients presented and how their disease was diagnosed. Study your patient's chart ahead of time and read the reports of all diagnostic procedures that have been performed, examine the blood work, and look up the pathology results of any biopsies. Make sure that you review the relevant imaging tests, not only by reading the written report, but also by looking at the actual pictures. Ask the resident who is assigned to the case to go over the films with you and point out the key findings. Once you have pieced together the patient's story and know the planned operation, review the relevant pathophysiology and study the anatomy for the procedure being performed.

Be sure to arrive at least 15 min before your case is scheduled to begin. Note that as the day progresses, the start time listed on the OR schedule is merely an estimate; cases will start earlier or later than the stated time, depending on whether the prior case has finished. In order to be on time for your assigned case you will have to keep track of whether the room is running on schedule. Once in the preoperative holding area, introduce yourself to your patient and ask

U. Sarpel, *Surgery: An Introductory Guide*,
DOI 10.1007/978-1-4939-0903-2_1,
© Springer Science+Business Media New York 2014

questions to fill in any gaps in your understanding of the history of illness.

Once your patient is brought into the operating room, it is a good idea to introduce yourself to both the circulating nurse and the scrub nurse. You should also introduce yourself to the attending surgeon if you have not met before. Help your resident with tasks like placing compression boots on your patient, inserting a urinary catheter, and shaving the operative site, as indicated. These may seem like small tasks, but they demonstrate your involvement and set the tone for rest of the case. Pay attention when the resident or attending performs a physical exam on your patient. Otherwise subtle findings often become evident once a patient is under anesthesia.

During the operation, stay focused and try to follow the sequence of events. In general, the more engaged you are, the more likely your team is to teach about the case. Most surgeons welcome thoughtful questions from a student during an operation, but make sure you do not ask any questions to which you should already know the answer. Be prepared to answer questions from your attending about the patient's history, the relevant anatomy, or the disease process at hand. If you do not know the answer to a question, the best response is usually "I'm not sure, but I'll look that up and get back to you."

At the completion of the operation, take the initiative to write the **brief operative note**. This exercise will ensure that you understood the particulars of the case, such as the name of the procedure, the estimated blood loss, and any unexpected complications. Discuss the **postoperative orders** with your resident so that you know which intravenous fluids, medications, and diet your patient will receive. A **postoperative check** is typically made on a patient 4–6 hours after surgery. Depending on your other clinical responsibilities, you should try to take part in this evaluation.

The operation may have ended, but your responsibility to the patient continues until their discharge home. Each morning, arrive early to check on your patients and gather the information you need to present on rounds with your surgical team. Surgical rounds tend to be fast paced and to the point. Practice delivering your presentation, and know your patient well enough that you can present without relying on notes. Although the preferred style varies, most surgical presentations follow the **SOAP** format: subjective, objective, assessment, and plan.

- The first sentence of a presentation is typically "(Patient name) is a (age) year-old (male/female), who is postoperative day (#) status-post a (procedure) for (disease process)."
- **Subjective**: This section begins with a brief summary of any significant overnight events such as fever, emesis, or chest pain. Next, describe any patient complaints such as adequacy of pain control, how the patient is tolerating their current diet, whether the patient has had any flatus or bowel movements, and if the patient has been ambulating. Limit this section to 1–2 sentences.
- **Objective**: The objective section begins with a statement of the vital signs and the fluid intake and output. The "ins" include the type and rate of intravenous fluid and parenteral or enteral nutrition that your patient is receiving. "Outs" include nasogastric tube output, urine output, and the amount of fluid in any surgical drains. It is also important to describe the quality of the fluid in drains; common descriptors of fluid quality are serous, serosanguinous, bilious, purulent, chylous, bloody, etc. The next portion of the objective section is the focused physical examination. Although your own morning exam should be thorough, on rounds it is usually acceptable to focus your presentation on the relevant body areas. The last portion of the objective section covers lab work. Rather than exhaustively listing every test, you should highlight a few relevant results such as white blood cell count, hematocrit, bilirubin, or any others that may be applicable to your patient's operation. Remember that

pertinent negatives can be as important as a positive finding.

- **Assessment**: Resist the urge to simply repeat your first sentence. The assessment section should be just that — your opinion on how the patient is doing. Use this portion to highlight any areas of concern you have about the patient's course and demonstrate your clinical judgement.
- **Plan**: For patients who are having an uneventful recovery, mention routine steps such as advancing the diet, discontinuing intravenous fluids, removing catheters and drains, or initiating discharge planning. In those patients who are experiencing a postoperative complication, describe how you will evaluate and treat the problem. For more complex patients, it may be useful to create a list of organ systems and provide an assessment and plan for each area.

You will be responsible for following your patients' postoperative course, and you should aim to be involved in every aspect of their medical care throughout their hospital stay. If your patient goes for an endoscopy, ask your team if you can observe; if your patient develops a complication and needs to return back to the operating room, you should make every effort to be present at the repeat surgery. By immersing yourself in your patient's care from beginning to end, you will learn a tremendous amount about their disease process. Finally, do not limit yourself to learning only about your own assigned patients. If there is another patient on the service with an interesting CT scan or physical exam finding, take the opportunity to gain from that experience as well.

Preparing for the OR

Preparation
- Ask to have your OR cases assigned the day before, so there is time to prepare
- Study the patient's medical records to understand the indications for surgery
- Presenting symptoms
- PMHx, PSHx
- Diagnostic work-up, including biopsies, procedures, blood work
- Imaging – review reports and images
- Review the pathophysiology of the patient's disease
- Study the anatomy relevant to the operation and the surgical field
- Understand the basic steps of the operation
- Know the most common complications of the operation

Patient interview
- Arrive in the holding area 15 minutes before the case starts
- Introduce yourself to your patient
- Ask questions to fill in any gaps in your understanding of the history
- Perform a focused physical exam

Prior to incision
- Introduce yourself to the nursing team
- Pull sterile gloves in your size
- Assist with compression boots, patient positioning, shaving incision site, and insertion of urinary catheter, as appropriate for case

After the case
- Write Brief Op Note
- Review post-op orders
- Perform a post-op check

Rounding

- You will be expected to pick-up each patient on whose operation you were scrubbed, and to follow them through their hospital stay
- Try to be involved with all aspects of your patient's medical care, including observing any procedures or tests
- Pre-round each morning to gather information for team rounds
- Assist with dressing changes as appropriate

Oral presentation

- (Patient name) is a (age)(gender) who is POD(#), s/p (operation), for (disease)
- Subjective: overnight events, pain control, diet, bowel function, ambulation
- Objective: vital signs, ins and outs, physical examination, lab results
- Assessment: describe patient's status
- Plan: list specific steps for the day such as awaiting bowel function, advancing diet, repleting electrolytes, fluid bolus, removal of drain, etc.

Suggested Readings

Deitch EA. Tools of the trade and rules of the road: a surgical guide. 1st ed. Philadelphia: Lippincott Williams & Wilkins; 1997. p. 275–80 [Chapter 29, Surgical Etiquette and Roundsmanship].

Blackbourne LH. Surgical recall. 6th ed. Philadelphia: Lippincott Williams & Wilkins; 2012. p. 1–31 [Chapter 1, Introduction].

2
Incisions

Introduction

With the advent of laparoscopy and other minimally invasive approaches, more and more operations can be performed through small incisions, thereby reducing the morbidity associated with large wounds. Nevertheless, there are instances where laparoscopy is either not feasible or would be unsafe, and an open incision is the best approach.

Several different types of incisions can be used to provide access to the body cavities. In the thorax, the most common incisions are a **sternotomy** and a **thoracotomy**. In the abdomen, the **vertical midline** incision is the most frequently used. Other options include a unilateral or bilateral **subcostal** (chevron) incision, a **paramedian** incision, or a **Pfannenstiel** incision. A **thoracoabdominal** incision is a single, large incision that spans both body cavities. Each incision has its own advantages and disadvantages; it is up to the surgeon to choose the route of entry that provides the best exposure for the intended operation while limiting morbidity to the patient.

Once the operation is complete, the phases of wound healing begin. Normal wound healing starts with an influx of neutrophils and macrophages that remove bacteria and devitalized tissue by phagocytosis. Next, fibroblasts migrate to the site and begin the work of collagen synthesis, angiogenesis, and re-epithelialization. With time, further remodeling and maturation of the wound occurs. Although the majority of the

U. Sarpel, *Surgery: An Introductory Guide*,
DOI 10.1007/978-1-4939-0903-2_2,
© Springer Science+Business Media New York 2014

healing process is complete at 6 weeks, the full strength and final appearance of a wound can take up to 1 year to be fully established.

Many factors contribute to wound healing and must be considered by the surgeon when planning surgery. Severe malnutrition, immunosuppression, recent chemotherapy, chronic steroid use, smoking, and diabetes are all associated with poor wound healing and higher rates of complications. To the degree possible, any such factors should be addressed prior to surgery in order to maximize the chance of normal healing. For example, in certain cases it may be advantageous to delay surgery in order to allow for a period of aggressive nutritional supplementation. In the postoperative period, attention to tight glycemic control in diabetics has been proven to reduce infectious complications.

Surgical Technique

The skin incision is made with a scalpel and carried down through the subcutaneous fat to the underlying fascia (Fig. 2.1). Once the fascia is reached, it is elevated and incised, taking care not to damage any underlying structures. Electrocautery should be used sparingly since necrotic fat promotes infection. When using a midline abdominal incision, it is important to accurately locate the **linea alba** where the fusion of the apo-neuroses of the abdominal muscles occurs (Fig. 2.2). Making the incision through the **decussation of fibers** avoids the rectus muscles and allows for a stronger fascial closure. For incisions that traverse muscle groups, slow electrocautery should be used to divide the muscle fibers and achieve hemostasis.

Upon completion of the operation, different techniques can be used to re-approximate the fascial edges. Typically a single running suture is used from both ends of the incision and tied together at the midpoint. Alternatively, multiple interrupted sutures can be used depending on the setting and surgeon preference. It is not necessary to suture together muscle or subcutaneous fat since the strength of a closure

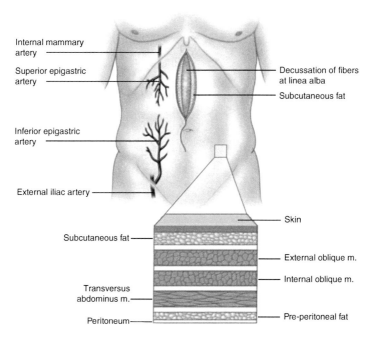

FIG. 2.1 Surgical anatomy for abdominal incisions: skin, subcutaneous fat, external oblique muscle, internal oblique muscle, transverses abdominus muscle, preperitoneal fat, peritoneum, decussation of fibers, linea alba, internal mammary artery, superior epigastric artery, external iliac artery, and inferior epigastric artery

comes from the fascia. In cases where the fascia is of too poor quality to hold sutures reliably, **retention sutures** can be used. These sutures are placed en masse through the skin and abdominal wall, and provide greater strength to maintain abdominal closure.

In certain situations, the fascia even can be temporarily left open. For example, if the patient is too unstable to remain in the OR, or if there is too much bowel edema present for the fascial edges to reach, then a **vacuum dressing** can be used. A sterile sponge is placed into the incision and covered

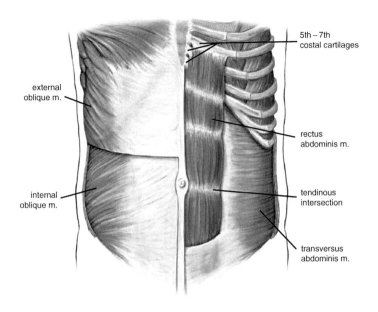

FIG. 2.2 Muscles of the anterior abdominal wall. [Reprinted from Prendergast PM. Anatomy of the Anterior Abdominal Wall. In: Shiffman M, Di Giuseppe A. Cosmetic Surgery: Art and Techniques. Heidelberg, Germany: Springer Verlag; 2013: 57-68. With permission from Springer Verlag.]

with a plastic sheet and is connected to a negative pressure machine. This dressing can be changed every 24–48 h, as needed and the fascial closure can be performed once patient has been stabilized or the bowel edema has resolved.

The skin itself can be closed primarily with sutures, surgical staples, or medical glue. In certain settings where there is not enough skin present to close a wound, alternative techniques can be used for coverage. Local **skin flaps** can be used to rotate or advance tissue into the surgical site and allow closure. A split or full-thickness **skin graft** can be taken from a separate body site and used to cover the wound. In order to survive, the skin graft must establish revascularization from the surgical bed. Therefore, skin grafts can only be used on clean wounds that have well-vascularized tissue present. Lastly, the skin may also be left open, in which case it will heal by **secondary intention**, a slow process where the wound contracts over a period of weeks. This approach is best for heavily soiled wounds.

An incision that is created and closed under sterile conditions is typically kept dressed until the second postoperative day. By that time, epithelialization across the wound is complete, effectively sealing it off from the outside world. After this time, the wound may be left uncovered, unless dressings are needed to absorb drainage, for patient comfort, or per surgeon preference.

The timing of removal of skin sutures or staples depends upon on the location of the incision. The face and neck heal very quickly, allowing for suture removal in as little as 3 days, whereas sutures in the abdomen and trunk are typically left in for at least 10 days. Sutures may need to be removed sooner to allow drainage if a wound infection is suspected.

Complications

Regardless of the size and location, all incisions carry the risk of **wound infection**. The topical application of sterilizing preps to the skin prior to incision destroys any bacteria present at the surface, however new bacteria migrate up from the intradermal glands within hours. Systemic antibiotics decrease the risk of wound infection and are given pre-incision in operations that involve contaminated areas such as the gastrointestinal or genitourinary tracts. It is important to re-dose antibiotics every few hours, as indicated, during a long operation.

Subcutaneous fat is poorly vascularized and provides ideal conditions for bacterial growth and abscess formation. Therefore, any postoperative erythema of the incision should be investigated for purulent collections by partially opening the skin and probing the subcutaneous fat. When operating in a grossly infected field (e.g., perforated appendicitis) the risk

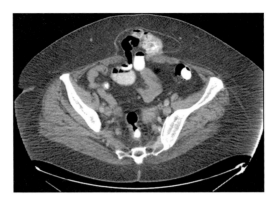

FIG. 2.3 CT scan image of a patient with an incisional hernia through a prior midline incision

of wound infection is so high, that the skin should be left open to allow for free drainage.

Dehiscence of the wound describes postoperative disruption of the fascia. This most often occurs secondary to a wound infection that has eroded away the underlying fascia allowing the sutures to pull through the tissue. The classic presentation of dehiscence is the new onset of copious salmon-colored fluid from the incision in the postoperative period. This fluid is normal peritoneal fluid that suddenly begins to drain through the wound once the fascial edges separate. Dehiscence can be accompanied by **evisceration** if the skin also opens and the abdominal viscera extrude through the wound. Patients may describe an incident of increased intra-abdominal pressure such as coughing or a bowel movement that resulted in a sudden opening of the incision with visible bowel. If evisceration occurs, immediate operative repair should be performed.

Longer-term issues with fascial healing can result in the patient developing an **incisional hernia** (Fig. 2.3). Most incisional hernias occur due to poor tissue strength, a technical error in closure, too much tension on the closure, or a postoperative wound infection. In addition, early resumption of physical activity can result in a hernia, and thus patients are advised to avoid heavy lifting for one month following surgery. Depending on the clinical scenario, most incisional hernias should be repaired due to the risk of incarceration and strangulation.

In the setting of trauma or sepsis, massive fluid resuscitation is sometimes required and can lead to extreme bowel edema. Forcibly closing the abdominal fascia over such edematous bowel causes elevated intra-abdominal pressures, known as **compartment syndrome**. These high pressures decrease perfusion to the kidneys, leading to oliguria and rising creatinine. In addition, intubated patients will demonstrate high peak airway pressures caused by the intra-abdominal organs compressing the diaphragms and limiting pulmonary capacity. The intra-abdominal pressure can be measured using a foley catheter equipped with a pressure transducer. If compartment syndrome is diagnosed, the abdominal fascia should be immediately opened to relieve the pressure.

Classic Case

A surgical consultation is requested on a 76-year-old diabetic, obese woman who presents with peritonitis. Evaluation with an upright chest X-ray reveals that she has free air under the diaphragm. Immediate operative exploration is performed through a vertical midline incision and reveals perforated diverticulitis with gross fecal contamination of the abdomen. A Hartmann's procedure is performed, where the proximal colon is exteriorized with a colostomy and a rectal stump is left in the pelvis. Antibiotics were administered prior to incision and are re-dosed appropriately throughout the operation. Upon completion of the operation, the fascia is closed with a running suture from either direction and the skin is only loosely approximated with staples.

The patient initially does well, but on the third postoperative day she develops a fever to 38.8 °C. Examination of the wound reveals blanching erythema of the skin with extension laterally across the abdominal wall. The staples at the site of greatest erythema are removed and probing of the wound is performed. The fascia is intact but some necrotic debris is present. Systemic antibiotics are initiated with some recession of the erythema and local wound care with twice-daily wet to dry dressing changes are initiated.

Two days later the surgical team is paged STAT by the nurse. While coughing, the patient suddenly felt a gush of fluid from her wound. On examination, the skin is open and small bowel is visible in the wound. The patient is urgently taken to the operating room. Inspection of the wound reveals poor healing and frankly necrotic fascia with loose sutures. The wound is closed with retention sutures. The patient ultimately has an uneventful recovery and is discharged home.

OR Questions

1. What patient factors are associated with poor wound healing?
   Obesity, advanced age, chronic steroid use, smoking, poor nutrition, diabetes, history of prior radiation, and early excessive physical activity.
2. What surgeon factors are associated with poor wound healing?
   Poor closure technique, excessive tension on the fascia inadequate administration of perioperative antibiotics, and inappropriate closure of a contaminated wound.
3. When closing an incision, is it advisable to suture together the layers of muscle and fat?
   No, sutures placed in muscle and fat add no strength to the wound. Only fascia provides the necessary integrity for wound closure.
4. Where are the majority of surgical site infections located?
   In the subcutaneous fat, between the skin and the fascia.
5. Can a wound infection be treated with antibiotics alone?
   No amount of antibiotics will cure a wound infection in the presence of an undrained purulent collection beneath the skin; opening the wound is the necessary treatment.

6. A patient with a well-healed scar from a previous paramedian incision now requires open surgery again. Is it advisable to make the incision through the previous scar, or to
   make a midline incision?

   *In general, the surgeon should choose the incision that best
   serves the needs of the current operation. However, it would
   be ideal to reuse the paramedian site, since a parallel incision may severely limit the blood supply to the area in
   between, risking tissue necrosis.*

Incisions

Vertical midline
- Most often used
- Minimal blood loss
- No division of muscle fibers
- No nerve injury
- Easy to open and close
- Good exposure to most abdominal and pelvic structures

Pfannenstiel
- Low transverse incision just above the pubis
- Excellent cosmetic results
- Exposure is limited to the pelvis

Subcostal
- Rectus muscle is divided, which can be more painful
- Provides exposure to gallbladder on the right, and spleen on the left
- A bilateral subcostal (chevron) incision offers excellent exposure to entire upper abdomen

Thoracic incisions
- Sternotomy: excellent exposure to the entire thoracic cavity, can be complicated by sternal wound infection
- Thoracotomy: provides access to each lung and the esophagus, can be used to clamp the aorta in trauma situations
- Thoracoabdominal: only used when necessary due to the morbidity associated with such a large incision

Paramedian
- Better exposure to lateral structures
- Lower incidence of incisional hernia because the abdomen is closed with multiple layers of fascia
- Costal margin limits vertical extension

Peri-op orders
- Pre-incision antibiotics for clean-contaminated or contaminated cases
- First dressing change for clean incisions is usually POD#2
- Infected incisions may need dressing changes bid, as indicated

Complications
- Infection: most wound infections are superficial to the facial closure: opening of the skin allows drainage and resolution
- Dehiscence: separation of the fascia, most often secondary to wound infection or excessive tension, may be heralded by the sudden new discharge of fluid from the wound
- Evisceration: protrusion of the abdominal viscera through the wound, due to a dehiscence, requires immediate operative repair
- Incisional hernia: essentially a late fascial dehiscence
- Compartment syndrome: elevated intra-abdominal pressure caused by closing the fascia in the setting of edematous bowel. May present with elevated creatinine or decreased urine output. A bladder pressure >25mmHg is diagnostic. Abdominal fascia must be opened for relief.

Suggested Readings

Roses RE, Morris JB. Incisions, closures, and management of the abdominal wound. In: Zinner MJ, Ashley SW, editors. Maingot's abdominal operations. 12th ed. New York: McGraw-Hill Professional Publishing; 2013.

Buck DW, Galiano RD. Wound care. In: Thorne CH, Chung KC, Gosain AK, Gurtner GC, Mehrara BJ, Rubin PJ, Spear SL, editors. Grabb and Smith's plastic surgery. 7th ed. Philadelphia: Lippincott Williams & Wilkins; 2014.

3
Laparoscopy

Introduction

In open surgery, an incision is made and the surgeon directly visualizes and handles the tissues in order to perform the operation. By contrast, laparoscopic surgery avoids a large incision by utilizing a camera and scope system to project images from within the body onto a monitor. A camera attached to a thin, long, lighted scope, and other instruments are inserted through small incisions, typically 1 cm or less in size. The positions of trocars are strategically chosen to provide the best approach to the area of interest. Once access to the abdomen is established, carbon dioxide is insufflated into the peritoneal cavity to create **pneumoperitoneum**. The insufflation pressure distends the abdominal wall outward, creating enough room for the surgeon to work. In the thoracic cavity, once the lung is deflated, the ribs maintain a rigid structure allowing thoracoscopy to be performed without insufflation.

Many if not most procedures that can be performed open can also be performed laparoscopically. In fact, for several operations such as cholecystectomy, appendectomy, and fundoplication, the laparoscopic approach has become the standard of care. Laparoscopic surgery carries the obvious advantage of smaller incisions and thus a more cosmetic postoperative appearance. However, numerous additional benefits to laparoscopy exist, including reduced postoperative

U. Sarpel, *Surgery: An Introductory Guide*,
DOI 10.1007/978-1-4939-0903-2_3,
© Springer Science+Business Media New York 2014

pain, fewer pulmonary complications, lower rates of wound infection, a shorter hospital stay, and fewer adhesions. Of note, the laparoscopic approach is strongly preferable in obese patients, since the morbidities associated with a large incision can be entirely avoided.

Despite the advantages afforded by laparoscopy, there are also certain disadvantages to this approach. In general, laparoscopy is technically more difficult and requires specialized training. In addition, laparoscopic cases carry risks unique to laparoscopy, including those related to trocar placement and pneumoperitoneum. Laparoscopy is not well suited to all patients; indeed, there are several instances where open surgery is advantageous. For example: (1) in trauma patients, rapid control of hemorrhage including direct manual compression of bleeding sites may be needed; (2) laparoscopy is difficult in the presence of extensive adhesions from previous operations or an intra-abdominal inflammatory process; (3) some patients with borderline pulmonary reserve cannot tolerate the reduced lung volumes caused by pneumoperitoneum and the resultant increased intrathoracic pressures; (4) the presence of extremely dilated bowel can make laparoscopy difficult since there is little room left to work; furthermore, dilated bowel is thin-walled and easily injured when grasped with laparoscopic instruments; and (5) when surgery is being performed for the resection of a large tumor, an incision may be necessary to extract the specimen.

Surgical Technique

The umbilicus is the most frequently used site to gain access to the abdomen, although other locations can also be used depending on the intended operation. The skin incision is made, the underlying fascia and peritoneum are opened, and a 1 cm **Hasson trocar** is placed through the hole. Rather than using this cut-down technique, percutaneous approaches are also available to gain access to the abdomen, and are used based on surgeon preference. Once the access has been established,

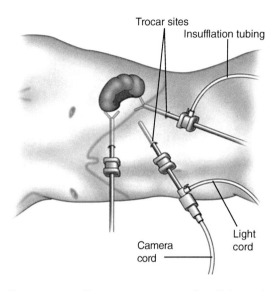

FIG. 3.1 Components of laparoscopy: trocar sites, light cord, camera cord, and insufflation tubing. Note the placement of trocars for triangulation around a target organ such as the spleen, and the use of positioning and gravity to optimize exposure

carbon dioxide is insufflated to create **pneumoperitoneum** to a pressure of approximately 15 mmHg. The camera is inserted into the abdomen and additional trocars are then placed under direct vision. The position, size, and number of port sites are carefully selected based on the type of operation being performed (Fig. 3.1).

Different types of scopes are available for laparoscopy. The most commonly used scopes are either 5 or 10 mm thick, and are available with varying degrees of angulation ($0°$, $30°$, and $45°$) to assist in visualizing around corners. New flexible scopes are also emerging onto the market. Throughout the case, the operating table can be tilted back and forth to allow gravity to assist in exposing target structures.

Specimens are typically placed within a plastic bag that is then pulled out the largest trocar site. The incision at this site may be enlarged slightly to facilitate removal. In certain cases (e.g., splenectomy) the specimen can be morcellated and removed piecemeal in order avoid enlarging the incision. After the operation is complete, the fascia of all port sites greater than 5 mm must be closed to prevent an incisional hernia.

Complications

In general, the complications of a laparoscopic operation are the same as for its open counterpart. However certain complications may be more common during laparoscopy. For example, the risk of **inadvertent enterotomy** may be greater for some types of laparoscopic surgery. Bowel may be injured during trocar placement—particularly during insertion of the first trocar since this is done with limited visualization.

An inadvertent enterotomy can also occur if a hot cautery appliance strays outside the visual field and touches a loop of intestine. An important concept in laparoscopic surgery is to maintain visualization of all instruments in order to avoid this complication. Finally, the limited sensory feedback in laparoscopic surgery can lead to situations where bowel is injured by rough handling.

In addition, some patients simply cannot tolerate the elevated intra-abdominal pressures that are created by insufflation. Patients with emphysema and limited pulmonary reserve may desaturate during longer laparoscopic procedures, in which case conversion to open surgery should occur. Similarly, the intra-abdominal pressures generated to achieve pneumoperitoneum cause a measurable decrease in the venous return to the heart, which can compromise the hemodynamics of patients with borderline cardiac output.

Classic Case

A 40-year-old woman with recurrent biliary colic undergoes a laparoscopic cholecystectomy. Access to the abdomen is established via a Hasson trocar inserted below the umbilicus. Pneumoperitoneum is created and three additional trocars are placed under direct vision. The procedure proceeds uneventfully, however the gallbladder contains a large stone that prevents removal of the specimen from the umbilical port site. The fascial incision at the site is enlarged slightly to allow removal of the gallbladder and stone. At the completion of the case, the umbilical trocar site is closed with a figure-of-eight suture. She is discharged home after a period of observation in the recovery room.

Five days postoperatively the patient presents to the emergency department complaining of persistent nausea and vomiting. In addition she states that she has not had any flatus or bowel movement in the past 2 days. On further questioning, the patient reports that a couple days ago she was lifting one of her children when she felt sudden pain at the umbilicus. On examination her abdomen is distended and tympanitic to percussion. The skin incisions at the trocar sites are all intact, but there is serosanguinous discharge from the umbilical port site.

A nasogastric tube is inserted with return of 800 cc of bilious fluid. A CT scan is performed which demonstrates loops of dilated small bowel with a transition zone at the level of the umbilical trocar site. The patient is taken back to the operating room, access to the abdomen is established through one of the prior trocar sites, and pneumoperitoneum is created. The dilated bowel loops are gently pushed aside to allow visualization. A segment of small intestine is seen herniating through the fascial incision at the umbilical trocar site. The figure-of-eight suture is seen to have torn through the fascia. The bowel is gently grasped and reduced back in the abdomen. Upon inspection, the bowel is edematous but pink and viable. The fascia at the site is carefully closed again. The patient makes an uneventful recovery, has return of bowel function, and is discharged home.

OR Questions

1. Following a laparoscopic cholecystectomy, a patient returns
   to the hospital with diffuse peritonitis. In the OR she is
   found to have enteric contents throughout the abdomen.
   What is the most likely cause?
   *An inadvertent enterotomy, caused either during trocar
   placement or by an unseen cautery injury to the bowel.*
2. A patient who needs a right hemicolectomy is requesting it
   be performed laparoscopically in order to reduce the risk
   of anastomotic leak. Is this correct?
   *While there are many benefits to laparoscopy, the rates of
   anastomotic leak are the same as in open surgery. It should
   always be emphasized that while the incisions are smaller,
   the surgery "on the inside" is still the same size.*
3. Toward the end of a laparoscopic appendectomy, the anesthesiologist reports crepitus around the patient's neck and
   face. What has occurred? What is the treatment?
   *Subcutaneous emphysema occurs when the pressurized gas
   leaks into the subcutaneous tissues and tracks along the
   fascial planes. It is generally harmless and resolves within
   days* (Fig. 3.2).
4. Durin the course of a long and difficult laparoscopic procedure, the anesthesiologist reports that the patient is
   developing progressively higher end-tidal CO_2 levels. What
   is the treatment?
   *The surgeon should consider converting to open surgery.
   The patient is likely unable to ventilate effectively due to the
   prolonged pneumoperitoneum which reduces the functional residual capacity and tidal volumes.*
5. The morning after a laparoscopic procedure, the patient
   complains of an aching pain in her shoulder. What is cause
   of this pain?
   *Residual pneumoperitoneum irritating the diaphragm
   causes referred pain to the shoulder. This is normal, and
   typically resolves within 2–3 days as the carbon dioxide is
   fully reabsorbed.*

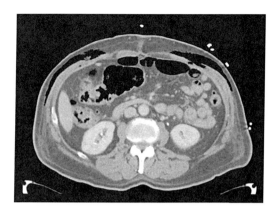

FIG. 3.2 CT scan image of a patient with extensive subcutaneous air following a laparoscopic procedure

6. A patient develops abdominal pain and fever 5 days after a laparoscopic ventral hernia repair. A CT scan demonstrates the presence of free air under the diaphragms. Is this normal?

No, the carbon dioxide from a laparoscopic procedure should be completely resorbed within the 3 days after surgery. The presence of significant free air 5 days after a laparoscopic procedure should raise the concern for bowel perforation.

Laparoscopy

Benefits
- Reduced post-operative pain
- Fewer pulmonary complications
- Lower rates of wound infection
- Smaller scar size
- Less adhesion formation

Limitations
- Contraindications include active hemorrhage, massively dilated bowel, dense adhesions
- Diagnostic laparoscopy can be used immediately prior to laparotomy to confirm intra-abdominal pathology

Hardware
- Camera
- Scope
    - straight (0°)
    - angled (30°, 45°)
- Light cord
- Insufflation tubing

Technique
- Establish pneumoperitoneum
    - Percutaneous (e.g. Veress needle)
    - Open (e.g. Hasson trocar)
- Insufflation with CO_2 to approximately 15 mmHg
- Position patient using gravity to maximize exposure to the area of interest
- Insert other trocars under direct vision
- Position and number of port sites are selected based on procedure

Complications
- Subcutaneous emphysema
- Low venous return and decreased tidal volumes secondary to increased intra-abdominal pressures
- Inadvertent enterotomy

Peri-op orders
- General anesthesia is required for sufficient relaxation of abdominal muscles
- Foley catheter should be placed if trocar placement near the bladder is anticipated
- Orders are generally the same as for the corresponding open operation

Suggested Readings

Jamal MK, Scott-Conner CEH. Patient selection and practical considerations in surgical endoscopy. In: Soper NJ, Swanström LL, Eubanks SW, Leonard ME, editors. Mastery of endoscopic and laparoscopic surgery: indications and techniques. 1st ed. Philadelphia: Lippincott Williams & Wilkins; 2009.

Katkhouda N. Advanced laparoscopic surgery: techniques and tips. 2nd ed. Berlin: Springer; 2010. p. 1–20 [Chapter 1, General Concepts].

4
Fundoplication

Introduction

Gastroesophageal reflux disease (GERD) occurs when an incompetent lower esophageal sphincter allows gastric acid to reflux into the esophagus, causing mucosal irritation. The classic symptom of GERD is a substernal burning pain that occurs after meals and is exacerbated by lying supine. Acid reflux can also cause respiratory symptoms such as coughing, laryngitis, and asthma-like wheezing secondary to aspiration. Because the symptoms of GERD are often nonspecific, the diagnosis may require a complement of tests including upper endoscopy, a barium swallow, esophageal manometry, and a 24-h pH test.

Over time, the persistent irritation caused by severe reflux can lead to the development of **Barrett's esophagus**, in which the normal squamous epithelium of the distal esophageal mucosa morphs into a glandular columnar epithelium. This process, known as intestinal metaplasia, can progress further into high-grade dysplasia and ultimately adenocarcinoma of the esophagus. Therefore the treatment of GERD serves to both relieve patient symptoms, and to lower the risk of future malignancy.

The treatment of GERD begins with lifestyle modifications such as advising patients to avoid foods that induce reflux, avoid eating before bedtime, elevate the head of the

U. Sarpel, *Surgery: An Introductory Guide*,
DOI 10.1007/978-1-4939-0903-2_4,
© Springer Science+Business Media New York 2014

bed, quit smoking, and lose excess body weight. Medications to treat GERD include H_2-blockers and proton-pump inhibitors. Surgical therapy for GERD is indicated when there is a failure of medical therapy to alleviate the symptoms, and/or the esophageal injury progresses to Barrett's esophagus. It is important to realize that in patients who are found to have high-grade dysplasia, invasive carcinoma is often also frequently present. Therefore an esophageal resection should be considered in patients with diffuse high-grade dysplasia.

GERD is sometimes associated with the presence of a **hiatal hernia**. A hiatal hernia occurs when the esophageal hiatus of the diaphragm is lax, and allows herniation of abdominal contents into the mediastinum. GERD and hiatal hernias are two separate diagnoses, which frequently coexist, although either can occur without the other. A **Type I** hernia, known as a sliding hiatal hernia, involves migration of only the GE junction into the chest. This change in location of the lower esophageal sphincter from the high pressure of the abdomen to the low pressure of the thorax can allow acid reflux to occur. Type I hernias are by far the most common kind of hiatal hernias, and are often discovered incidentally. As in other patients with GERD, treatment of individuals with Type I hiatal hernias is with medical therapy first, and surgical fundoplication as needed.

In a **Type II**—or paraesophageal—hernia, the GE junction remains in the abdomen, but the fundus of the stomach herniates up into the thorax. A **Type III** hernia is a combination of Types I and II, where both the GE junction and the fundus are in the chest (Fig. 4.1). Finally, in **Type IV** hernias, herniation of the stomach is accompanied by other organs such as the colon or the spleen (Fig. 4.2). Hernia Types II–IV are distinct from Type I hernias in that the herniated portion of bowel is at risk for becoming acutely incarcerated and strangulated. Therefore, all patients who are discovered to have a Type II–IV hernia should undergo surgical repair upon diagnosis, even if asymptomatic.

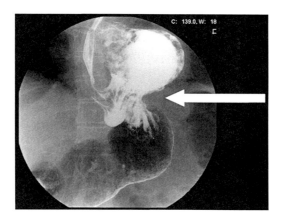

FIG. 4.1 Upper GI series demonstrating a Type III hiatal hernia; note the indentation of the diaphragmatic hiatus on the stomach (*arrow*), and that both the GE junction and the fundus are located in the thoracic cavity

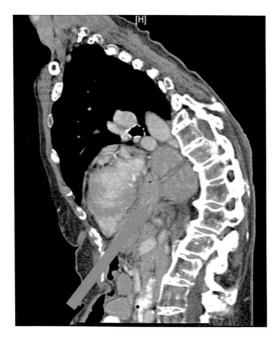

FIG. 4.2 Sagittal CT scan images of a patient with a large Type IV hiatal hernia; note the retrocardiac herniation of small bowel

Surgical Technique

Surgical therapy for GERD aims to decrease reflux by physically reinforcing the lower esophageal sphincter. A fundoplication procedure uses the fundus of the stomach to create a wrap around the lower esophagus, thereby increasing the pressure at the sphincter (Fig. 4.3). This procedure also alters the angle of the GE junction which may contribute to its antireflux effect. A laparoscopic **Nissen fundoplication** is the most common type of wrap currently performed. It involves using the fundus of the stomach to wrap 360° around the esophagus. Different types of fundoplication vary by the completeness of the wrap, and by whether a transabdominal or transthoracic approach is used.

In order to perform a Nissen fundoplication, the esophagus and stomach must be fully mobilized to allow for the wrap to reach circumferentially around the esophagus. The lesser sac is entered between the stomach and the greater omentum. This opening is propagated laterally until the **short gastric arteries** are encountered. These vessels are serially

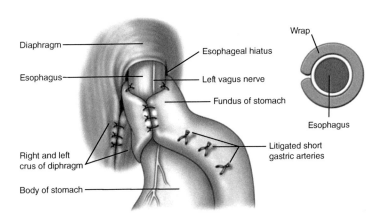

Fig. 4.3 Surgical anatomy for Nissen fundoplication: diaphragm, esophageal hiatus, right/left crus, esophagus, gastric fundus, vagus nerve, and short gastric arteries

divided along the length of the greater curvature until the GE junction is reached. Excessive traction on the stomach can lead to tearing of these fragile vessels resulting in significant hemorrhage.

Next, the lesser omentum between the liver and the stomach is opened, exposing the **diaphragmatic crus** and the **esophageal hiatus**. At this point the **vagus nerves** should be identified and protected. The esophagus is dissected away from the crura and other attachments until the distal portion is brought down into the abdomen. A rubber drain is placed around the esophagus to facilitate its manipulation.

The fully mobilized fundus of the stomach is passed posterior to the esophagus, and wrapped around to the front. The wrap should be sufficiently tension-free such that it will remain in this position even before the placement of tacking sutures. Also, it is important to ensure that the wrap sits on the esophagus itself, rather than on the body of the stomach. Prior to completing the fundoplication, the esophageal hiatus is closed by approximating the diaphragmatic crura with interrupted sutures. Finally, the wrap is sutured into place over a bougie in order to ensure that it is not made too tight.

The technique to repair a Type II–IV hiatal hernia begins with reducing the herniated organs into the abdomen, thus reestablishing normal anatomy. Next, the diaphragmatic defect is closed to prevent recurrence. Depending on the size of the defect, either the diaphragmatic crura can be sutured together as described above, or a piece of synthetic mesh can be used. A fundoplication is typically added to the procedure to treat any accompanying GERD, and to anchor the GE junction and stomach below the diaphragm.

Complications

During dissection around the GE junction, an **inadvertent enterotomy** into either the esophagus or the stomach can occur. It is crucial to recognize this injury intraoperatively in order to prevent significant morbidity from a leak. If an injury is identified, the perforation is closed primarily and the fundal wrap is placed over the repair in order to buttress it. Another potential complication is a **pneumothorax**, which can occur if the pleural space is entered during dissection of the mediastinum.

Dysphagia is a relatively common occurrence after fundoplication. Patients may also complain of **gas-bloat syndrome** which describes the uncomfortable feeling of not being able to burp. Dysphagia and bloating are usually due to edema at the wrap, and typically resolve within a week. However, persistent dysphagia may indicate that the wrap is too tight and may warrant surgical revision.

A **slipped wrap** develops when part of the stomach slides up through the wrap, above the fundoplication. Patients with this complication will complain of a recurrence of their heartburn. Slippage can occur either immediately in the postoperative period, or develop gradually over months. Operative revision is necessary to correct this complication.

Classic Case

A 46-year-old man presents to his primary care doctor complaining of several years of heartburn. He reports that his symptoms have not been effectively relieved despite dietary modifications and medical therapy with a proton-pump inhibitor. He is referred to a gastroenterologist who performs an upper endoscopy that demonstrates Barrett's esophagus. Several biopsies of the distal esophagus are taken and do not reveal dysplasia. 24-h pH monitoring confirms acid reflux into the distal esophagus correlating with the patient's symptoms. Esophageal manometry confirms normal esophageal motility, and a barium swallow study demonstrates the presence of a Type I hiatal hernia.

Given his persistent symptoms despite medical therapy, he is referred to a surgeon who performs an uncomplicated Nissen fundoplication. On postoperative day #1 a clear liquid diet is started, but the patient reports feeling bloated with difficulty swallowing. The patient is kept NPO with intravenous fluid hydration. Over the next several days, the patient's symptoms abate and he is able to tolerate liquids. Ultimately, his diet is advanced and he is discharged home.

OR Questions

1. What dietary modifications may be effective in reducing acid reflux?
   Caffeine, spicy foods, and alcohol are all known to exacerbate GERD symptoms; avoiding these may provide symptom relief.

2. What are the presenting signs and symptoms of a strangulated hiatal hernia?
   Patients typically complain of sudden chest or abdominal pain that is usually accompanied by nausea and retching. The diagnosis is confirmed by a CT scan which will demonstrate the herniation. A high degree of suspicion is required to make this diagnosis promptly since the signs and symptoms can be non-specific, and most patients are unaware that they have a hiatal hernia.

3. On POD#1 following a Nissen fundoplication a patient becomes tachycardic to 105 bpm and has a fever of 38.8 °C. What is the clinical concern?
   The patient may have a leak from an inadvertent injury to the stomach. An emergent UGI with gastrograffin may be used to determine if a leak is present. If the clinical suspicion is sufficiently high, the surgeon may choose to re-explore the patient without any imaging.

4. A patient with long-standing GERD is taken for a Nissen fundoplication. During the dissection of the distal esophagus the surgeon notices billowing of the left diaphragm and the anesthesiologist reports that she is suddenly having difficulty maintaining the patient's oxygen saturation. What is the diagnosis and treatment?
   Auscultation will confirm the presence of a pneumothorax. The surgeon should desufflate the abdomen and observe for

resolution of the hypoxia. Any hemodynamic instability should prompt the immediate placement of a chest tube.

5. A patient involved in a motor vehicle collision complains of shortness of breath. Decreased breath sounds are noted on auscultation of the left chest. In addition to pneumothorax, what should be included in the differential diagnosis?

*Significant blunt force impact can lead to **diaphragmatic rupture** with resultant herniation of abdominal contents into the thoracic cavity.*

Fundoplication

Gastroesophageal reflux disease (GERD)

- Decreased pressure at the lower esophageal sphincter allows reflux of acidic gastric contents into the distal esophagus
- Often asymptomatic, or may present with heartburn, regurgitation, dysphagia, laryngitis, hoarseness, cough
- Barrett's esophagus: change in the esophageal mucosa from its usual squamous to a columnar epithelium, increases the risk of adenocarcinoma
- Evaluation involves endoscopy, manometry, pH monitoring, and upper GI imaging

Hiatal hernia

- Occurs when structures herniate through a lax esophageal hiatus up into the mediastinum
- Type I: herniation of only GE junction
- Type II: herniation of the fundus of the stomach
- Type III: a combination of Type I and Type II
- Type IV: herniation of other organs (e.g. spleen, colon)
- Non-operative therapy is used for type I hernias
- Hiatal hernia repair is usually recommended for types II-IV, since incarceration and strangulation of hernia contents can occur

Technique
- Nissen fundoplication is most common technique
- Usually performed laparoscopically
- Dissection of the esophageal hiatus
- Ligation of short gastric arteries and mobilization of the stomach fundus
- Approximation of diaphragmatic crura to tighten esophageal hiatus
- Fundus is wrapped around the esophagus and sutured in place
- May be performed with hiatal hernia repair as needed

Peri-op orders
- Antiemetic agents
- Consider post-op upper GI study
- Clear liquids on POD#1
- Advance diet as tolerated

Complications
- Enterotomy
- Pneumothorax
- Dysphagia
- Gas-bloat syndrome
- Slipped wrap

Suggested Reading

Linden PA. Overview: esophageal reflux disorders. In: Sugarbaker DJ, Bueno R, Krasna MJ, Mentzer SJ, Zellos L, editors. Adult chest surgery. 1st ed. New York: McGraw-Hill Professional Publishing; 2009.

5
Esophagectomy

Introduction

Resection of the esophagus is most commonly performed for
the treatment of esophageal carcinoma. Two histologic sub-
types of this cancer exist, each with their own distinctive
features. Worldwide, by far the most common type of esophageal cancer is **squamous cell carcinoma** (SCC). This tumor
type is associated with smoking and alcohol intake, which are
individual risk factors for SCC and also have a synergistic
effect when combined. While rates of SCC in other countries
remain high, over the past few decades the incidence in the
USA has been steadily dropping—a change attributed to
lower rates of tobacco and alcohol use.

At the same time, there has been a dramatic rise in the
incidence of **esophageal adenocarcinoma**, such that adenocarcinoma has recently surpassed squamous cell carcinoma
as the most common type of esophageal cancer in the USA.
Esophageal adenocarcinoma is thought to occur as the end
result of a sequence of events that culminate in carcinogen-
esis. The first step in this process is the development of
gastroesophageal reflux disease (GERD), in which a lax
lower esophageal sphincter allows acidic contents of the
stomach to reflux into the lower esophagus. Chronic irritation
from GERD can lead to transformation of the normal strati-
fied squamous epithelium of the esophagus into a columnar
epithelium, a change known as intestinal metaplasia—or

Barrett's esophagus. With continued insult, these columnar cells can become dysplastic, and may ultimately undergo malignant degeneration into adenocarcinoma. The rise in rates of adenocarcinoma in the USA can in part be explained by the prevalence of obesity and associated GERD.

Patients diagnosed with GERD should be treated with medications and anti-reflux surgery, as indicated, in order to reduce acid reflux and prevent subsequent intestinal metaplasia. Once a diagnosis of Barrett's esophagus has been established, patients should be monitored closely with endoscopy and random esophageal biopsies. Most patients with mild dysplasia will never go on to develop esophageal cancer, however if **high-grade dysplasia** is present on biopsies, there is a significant chance of carcinoma being present elsewhere in unsampled areas of the esophagus. For this reason, the presence of high-grade dysplasia is in itself considered an indication for esophagectomy. However, newer approaches to the treatment of high-grade dysplasia and carcinoma in situ are emerging, including photodynamic therapy, endoscopic mucosal resection, and thermal ablation of affected areas. These approaches offer less invasive alternatives to esophagectomy and appear to have favorable results in appropriately selected patients.

Unfortunately, most patients with esophageal cancer present with advanced disease. Typical symptoms at presentation are progressive dysphagia and unintentional weight loss. Any patient presenting with these complaints should undergo upper endoscopy for evaluation. If esophageal cancer is discovered, an endoscopic ultrasound is performed to assess the tumor depth (**T stage**) and to look for suspicious appearing lymph nodes (**N stage**). A CT scan is obtained to visualize the tumor's relationship to adjacent structures and to assess for distant metastatic disease (Fig. 5.1). PET is very useful in evaluating for metastatic disease, since esophageal cancer tends to be highly metabolic and thus glucose-avid (Fig. 5.2).

The minority of individuals who present with early stage disease may proceed directly to surgical resection. However, the majority of patients will have locally advanced disease

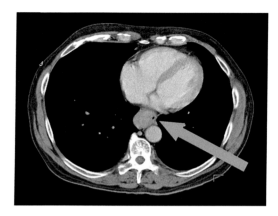

FIG. 5.1 Axial CT scan image of a patient with esophageal carcinoma. Note the eccentric wall thickening and compressed, displaced lumen of the esophagus

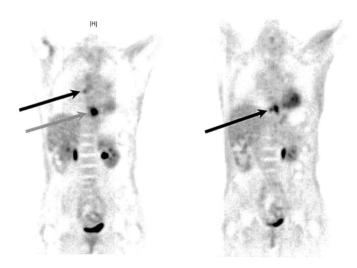

FIG. 5.2 PET images of a patient with esophageal carcinoma demonstrating the glucose-avid primary tumor (*blue arrow*) and adjacent lymphadenopathy (*black arrows*); note the normal physiologic uptake in the myocardium, kidneys, and bladder

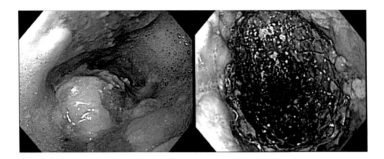

FIG. 5.3 Endoscopic view of a near-obstructing esophageal squamous cell cancer before and after stent placement

and are typically treated with **neoadjuvant chemoradiation** therapy prior to surgery.

Presurgical nutritional optimization is an important component of the treatment of a patient with esophageal carcinoma. **Endoscopic stent** placement can be a useful method of relieving the dysphagia that patients have due to the mass effect of the tumor (Fig. 5.3). This minimally invasive procedure allows patients to resume oral intake and maximize their nutritional status. If stent placement is not feasible, a jejunostomy tube can be used for enteral feeding during treatment. Gastrostomy tubes should be generally avoided since the stomach may be used as the future reconstructive conduit. Placement of a jejunostomy tube is described in detail in the section on enteral access.

Squamous cell carcinoma of the esophagus is significantly more chemoresponsive than adenocarcinoma, and some patients undergoing neoadjuvant therapy will achieve complete remission of their tumor. It is now increasingly accepted that these complete responders do not require esophagectomy. Such patients are closely observed for signs of recurrence, at which point surgery can be reconsidered. Unlike squamous cell carcinoma, patients with adenocarcinoma rarely achieve complete response to neoadjuvant therapy, and surgical resection is nearly always required.

Although less common, esophageal surgery is also occasionally indicated for nonmalignant etiologies. Ingestion of bleach,

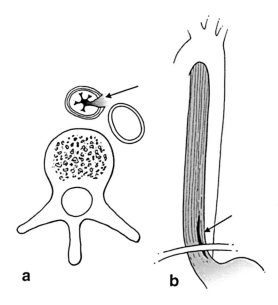

FIG. 5.4 Illustration of Boerhaave's syndrome, demonstrating the most common site of perforation along the left-posterior aspect of the distal esophagus [Reprinted from Restrepo CS, Lemos DF, Ocazionez D, et al. Intramural hematoma of the esophagus: a pictorial essay. Emergency Radiology 2008; 15(1):13-22. With permission from Springer Verlag]

lye, or other caustic agents causes chemical burns to the esophagus, resulting in stricture formation. Esophageal resection and reconstruction may be indicated for severe cases.

Traumatic rupture of the esophagus—known as **Boerhaave's syndrome**—can occur from violent retching, typically following excessive consumption of food and alcohol. Classic signs of a Boerhaave's perforation include chest pain, fever, tachypnea, and tachycardia, associated with a left pleural effusion and mediastinal emphysema. The most common site of tearing is along the left-posterior aspect of the distal esophagus (Fig. 5.4). Perforation of the esophagus can also result from iatrogenic injury during upper endoscopy, most often during dilation of esophageal strictures.

Prompt diagnosis is key to the management of these traumatic injuries. If there is a suspicion of perforation, an esophagram using water-soluble contrast should be obtained immediately. If the injury is diagnosed within 24 h, it is usually possible to perform a primary repair of the defect. However, if diagnosis is delayed, the ensuing infection and inflammation cause the surrounding tissues to become friable and not amenable to suture repair. In these cases, esophageal diversion with wide drainage, and staged reconstruction may be necessary.

Surgical Technique

Multiple approaches to the esophagus are possible, and selection of technique is dependent on tumor location, depth of invasion, and surgeon preference. Most procedures are variations on either the Ivor-Lewis transthoracic esophagectomy or the transhiatal esophagectomy, both of which are described in detail here.

An **Ivor-Lewis esophagectomy** combines a laparotomy incision with a right thoracotomy. The operation begins with an abdominal incision, where the stomach is fashioned into a conduit to replace the esophagus. In order to reach into the thoracic cavity, the stomach and duodenum must be extensively mobilized, requiring that all gastric arteries except the right gastroepiploic be ligated. The stomach has a robust 360° blood supply from the paired right and left gastric and gastro-epiploic arteries, and adequate perfusion of the entire organ can be maintained even with ligation of three of these four blood vessels.

When the esophagus is resected, the vagus nerves are also transected; this causes denervation of the pylorus and can lead to gastric outlet obstruction. Depending on surgeon preference, a pyloromyotomy or pyloroplasty is usually performed during preparation of the gastric conduit to avoid this complication. Once the abdominal portion of the operation is complete, the laparotomy incision is closed and dressed.

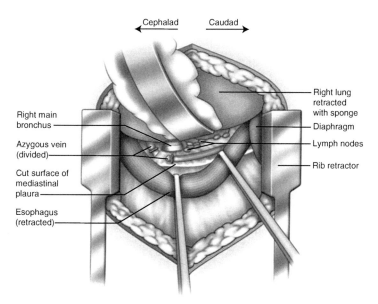

Cephalad   Caudad

Right main bronchus

Azygous vein (divided)

Cut surface of mediastinal plaura

Esophagus (retracted)

Right lung retracted with sponge

Diaphragm

Lymph nodes

Rib retractor

FIG. 5.5 Surgical anatomy during Ivor-Lewis esophagectomy: right lung, right main bronchus, mediastinal pleura, azygous vein, thoracic esophagus, and diaphragm

The patient is then turned into a lateral decubitus position and a right thoracotomy is performed through the fifth intercostal space (Fig. 5.5). The right lung is collapsed and reflected out of the field. The mediastinal pleura is then opened along the length of the esophagus, to allow for access and mobilization. The esophagus and tumor are carefully dissected away from the mediastinum.

The proximal esophagus is transected and the prepared gastric conduit is pulled up into the thoracic cavity. The distal transection is made just below the GE junction, freeing the esophageal specimen. Next, a complete thoracic lymphadenectomy is performed. One of the benefits of the Ivor-Lewis is that this approach allows for direct visualization of the tumor and permits an en bloc resection with surrounding tissues, including the regional lymph nodes. The stomach is then fashioned into a tubular shape to create a neo-esophagus. An anastomosis is made between the proximal esophageal remnant and the gastric conduit. This can be performed in a stapled or hand-sewn manner. Chest tubes are left in the thorax and the incision is closed.

A **transhiatal esophagectomy** is performed via a laparotomy and a left neck incision; no thoracotomy is performed in this type of esophagectomy. The mobilization of the stomach is performed in the same manner as previously described. However, instead of a thoracotomy to approach the esophagus, the surgeon uses blunt manual dissection up the mediastinum, gently freeing the esophagus from its attachments in all directions.

An oblique left neck incision is made along the anterior border of the sternocleidomastoid muscle. The proximal esophagus is identified and divided, allowing the esophagus to be pulled down into the abdomen. The transection of the stomach and construction of the gastric conduit are the same as previously described. The tubularized stomach is delivered up through the mediastinal tunnel towards the neck. The gastroesophageal anastomosis is then performed through the neck incision, in either a stapled or hand-sewn fashion.

One benefit of the transhiatal esophagectomy is that a more proximal margin on the esophagus can be obtained than by a right thoracotomy. In addition, the pain and morbidity of the thoracic incision are avoided. However, because of the relatively blind nature of the dissection, this approach can only be used for smaller tumors that do not invade surrounding structures. Another disadvantage is the lack of formal thoracic lymphadenectomy. Some of the pros and cons of these approaches can be modified with a three-incision esophagectomy, which utilizes a cervical, thoracic, and abdominal approach.

All of the above described esophagectomy procedures can be further augmented using minimally invasive techniques in either the abdominal and/or thoracic portions. Laparoscopic and thoracoscopic techniques help limit the incision-related complications of esophagectomy.

Depending on the situation, placement of a jejunal feeding tube should be considered to ensure excellent nutrition during the postoperative period. In the event of a leak at the esophageal anastomosis, enteral nutrition can continue uninterrupted via the jejunostomy tube, while the anastomosis is allowed to heal.

Complications

As in other gastrointestinal resections, the most serious complication of an esophagectomy is an **anastomotic leak**. The incidence and treatment of this complication differs significantly depending on what type of reconstruction was performed.

With an Ivor-Lewis esophagectomy, the anastomosis is performed in the thoracic cavity. The benefit of this approach is that the gastric conduit need only reach up to the point of esophageal transection in the chest. As a result, there is little tension on the anastomosis and the blood supply to the gastric conduit is under less stretch. Both the lack of tension and the robust tissue perfusion explain the lower leak rate associated with an Ivor-Lewis esophagectomy. Unfortunately, although the chance of a leak is less, the complications of a leak when it does occur are significantly higher. When an anastomotic leak occurs within the thoracic cavity, the spillage of enteric contents leads to an intense mediastinitus, often resulting in empyema and significant morbidity.

In a transhiatal esophagectomy, the anastomosis of the gastric conduit to the esophagus is performed through a cervical incision. As a result, the stomach must be pulled up to the level of the neck, and the anastomosis may be under some degree of tension. In addition, the blood supply to the tip of the gastric conduit may be attenuated due to the greater distance and stretch on the tissues. The leak rate of a cervical anastomosis is generally higher than a thoracic anastomosis, however the sequelae of a cervical leak are significantly less since the contamination is limited to the subcutaneous tissues of the neck. Opening the neck incision to allow the enteric contents to drain is usually sufficient to allow the leak to heal.

Once the acute inflammation of an anastomotic leak resolves, stricture formation at the anastomosis is a likely consequence. Fortunately most **anastomotic strictures** can be handled satisfactorily with serial endoscopic dilations. Surgical revision of the anastomosis is rarely required. Stricture formation which develops long after the postoperative period should raise the suspicion of local tumor recurrence, and should be investigated with imaging and endoscopic biopsies.

Classic Case

A 67-year-old man with a history of GERD presents with progressive dysphagia. He is able to tolerate liquids and soft foods, but over the past 3 months reports a 25 lbs weight loss. Upper endoscopy reveals a distal esophageal stricture and biopsies demonstrate adenocarcinoma in the setting of Barrett's esophagus. On CT scan of the chest and abdomen there are no distant metastases present. A PET scan demonstrates a highly glucose-avid primary tumor in the distal esophagus and regional lymphadenopathy. Endoscopic ultrasound is performed and a uT3N1 tumor is diagnosed. He undergoes nutritional counseling and begins taking high-calorie dietary supplements.

The patient then receives neoadjuvant treatment with chemotherapy and radiation, which he tolerates without incident. After completing this regimen, imaging reevaluation demonstrates no new metastases and moderate regression of the primary tumor and regional nodes. An Ivor-Lewis esophagectomy is performed without intraoperative complications. A postoperative esophagram reveals a patent anastomosis without evidence of a leak. His diet is advanced and the surgical drains are removed. He is discharged home and once recovered resumes adjuvant chemotherapy with close surveillance for recurrence.

OR Questions

1. What is the clinical significance of voice hoarseness in a patient who is diagnosed with esophageal cancer?
   Tumor involvement of the recurrent laryngeal nerve.
2. Where along the esophagus is adenocarcinoma most commonly found and why?
   The pathophysiology of its development from GERD explains why esophageal adenocarcinoma is most commonly found in the lower third of the esophagus, whereas squamous cell carcinoma typically occurs in the upper and middle portions of the esophagus.
3. Do all patients with esophageal adenocarcinoma carry a prior diagnosis of GERD?
   No. Although adenocarcinoma of the esophagus can arise from a region of Barrett's esophagus as a result of acid reflux, it is important to note that many patients diagnosed with esophageal adenocarcinoma do not describe a history of reflux symptoms.
4. What organs can be used for the reconstructive conduit?
   Although the stomach is the preferred conduit, a segment of the colon or the jejunum can also be used for reconstruction if the stomach is not suitable.
5. What noninvasive options are available for a patient with outlet obstruction of the gastric conduit following esophagectomy?
   Outlet obstruction is typically due to spasm of the pyloric muscle, and can occur with incomplete pyloromyotomy. Endoscopic injection of botulinum toxin into the pylorus will paralyze the muscle and allow passage of gastric contents.
6. If an anastomotic leak is suspected after an Ivor-Lewis esophagectomy, what test can be performed on the fluid from the chest tubes?
   The presence of amylase in the fluid from the thoracic drains suggests an anastomotic leak.

Esophagectomy

Esophageal carcinoma
- Adenocarcinoma: increasing incidence, associated with obesity and GERD, arises from a background of Barrett's esophagus, in distal third of esophagus
- Squamous cell carcinoma: associated with smoking and alcohol intake, usually in upper or middle third of esophagus
- Symptoms include reflux, dysphagia, weight loss

Evaluation
- Upper endoscopy with biopsy
- Endoscopic ultrasound
- CT scan
- PET scan
- Bronchoscopy if invasion into bronchus is suspected

Treatment
- Neoadjuvant chemoradiation if locally advanced
- Esophagectomy
- Adjuvant chemotherapy
- Squamous cell carcinoma may have complete response to neoadjuvant therapy, and may not require resection

Benign indications
- Stricture: ingestion of caustic materials can cause chemical burns that lead to stricture
- Boerhaave's syndrome: perforation of the esophagus caused by severe retching

Technique: Transhiatal resection
- Laparotomy with mobilization of stomach and pyloromyotomy
- Blunt manual dissection of esophagus from abdomen upwards
- Left neck incision, division of proximal esophagus
- Esophagus brought down into the abdomen and resected
- Preparation of gastric conduit
- Gastroesophageal anastomosis is performed in the neck
- Consider feeding jejunostomy
- May have higher rate of anastomotic leak than transthoracic approach, however leaks are associated with less morbidity and rarely require reoperation

Technique: Ivor-Lewis esophagectomy
- Laparotomy with mobilization of stomach and pyloromyotomy
- Consider feeding jejunostomy
- Right thoracotomy, resection of esophagus with lymphadenectomy
- Preparation of gastric conduit
- Anastomosis in the chest
- Lower rate of anastomotic leak, but higher risk of mediastinitus and mortality if leak occurs

Complications
- Anastomotic leak: may be due to ischemia and/or tension on anastomosis
- Anastomotic stricture

Peri-op orders
- NPO/NGT
- Consider upper GI study to assess anastomosis
- Initiate feeds if J-tube placed

Suggested Readings

Li CM, McCoy JA, Hsu HK. Esophagus. In: Lawrence PF, editor. Essentials of general surgery. 5th ed. Philadelphia: Lippincott Williams & Wilkins; 2013.

Krasna M, Ebright M. Overview: esophageal and proximal stomach malignancy. In: Sugarbaker DJ, Bueno R, Krasna MJ, Mentzer SJ, Zellos L, editors. Adult chest surgery. 1st ed. New York: McGraw-Hill Professional Publishing; 2009.

6
Gastrectomy

Introduction

Gastric surgery may be indicated for a wide variety of benign or malignant conditions. In the past, the most frequent reason for an operation on the stomach was **peptic ulcer disease**. With the advent of proton-pump inhibitors and therapy for *H. pylori* medical management has largely replaced surgical treatment for this disease. Nevertheless, patients still occasionally present with complications of ulcer disease requiring surgery such as free air from a perforation (Fig. 6.1), bleeding ulcer, or pyloric stricture. In patients who have never tried pharmacologic therapy, it is best to simply address the surgical emergency and initiate proton-pump therapy postoperatively. However, patients who are truly refractory to medical therapy may benefit from an antrectomy and vagotomy to decrease acid production. ᴸᴰ remove ᴸᴰ remove antrum part of vagus

The object of surgical therapy of peptic ulcer disease is to block the two agents that most stimulate acid secretion by the parietal cell: **gastrin** and **acetylcholine**. The antrum of the stomach is the region that contains G-cells that secrete gastrin into the systemic circulation; the goal of antiacid surgery is to resect the antrum, and thus eliminate the source of gastrin. The other mechanism driving acid secretion by the parietal cells is acetylcholine, which is released via vagal nerve stimulation. A **truncal vagotomy** involves ligating the main right and left vagal trunks that lie along the esophagus.

U. Sarpel, *Surgery: An Introductory Guide*,
DOI 10.1007/978-1-4939-0903-2_6,
© Springer Science+Business Media New York 2014

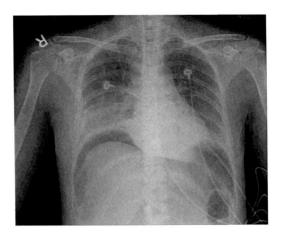

FIG. 6.1 Upright chest X-ray of a patient with free intra-abdominal air secondary to a perforated ulcer

The combination of antrectomy and vagotomy thereby dramatically reduces acid production and allows healing of the gastric or duodenal ulcer.

It is important to keep in mind that not every ulcer is acid related. Atypical ulcers, such as those located in the proximal stomach, or non-healing ulcers, should raise suspicion for an underlying malignancy and should be biopsied for further evaluation. Indeed, **gastric adenocarcinoma** is now the leading indication for gastrectomy (Fig. 6.2). Major risk factors for the development of gastric cancer include *Helicobacter pylori* infection, Asian ethnicity, smoking, a diet high in cured meats, and pernicious anemia. Interestingly, a history of prior partial gastrectomy also confers a greater risk for gastric adenocarcinoma, known as **gastric remnant cancer**. Gastric cancer is usually insidious in onset, and patients do not become symptomatic until the disease is relatively advanced.

Once a clinical suspicion of cancer exits, upper endoscopy and biopsy are performed for diagnosis. Next, a CT scan is obtained to evaluate for metastatic disease, most often found in the liver. Gastric cancer also has a predilection for early peritoneal dissemination, and a diagnostic laparoscopy should

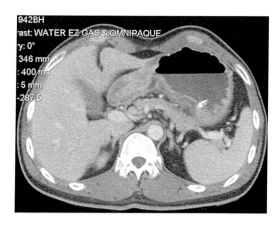

FIG. 6.2 CT scan image of a patient with a gastric adenocarcinoma in the antrum; note the normal proximal stomach in comparison to the thick-walled, non-distensible distal stomach

be performed to rule out **carcinomatosis**. If no metastases are present, then patients are candidates for surgical resection. Prior to surgery, many centers include **endoscopic ultrasound** (**EUS**), in their staging work-up. If the tumor is deep (**T stage** ≥3) or there is evidence of nodal involvement (**N stage** ≥1), neoadjuvant chemotherapy is administered prior to resection.

Gastric adenocarcinomas have a tendency for submucosal spread that is always more extensive than suggested by the gross size of the tumor. Therefore surgical resection must include 6 cm margins beyond the visible extent of the tumor. Interestingly, margins need not extend past the esophagus or the pylorus, since these sphincters act as natural barriers to tumor extension. A lymph node dissection should be included in the procedure, although the extent of lymphadenectomy required is somewhat controversial. While the literature on the subject is mixed, many centers advocate a modified **D2 lymphadenectomy**. This dissection includes resection of the perigastric nodes as well as a dissection of the lymph nodes along the celiac trunk, common hepatic artery, left gastric artery, and splenic artery.

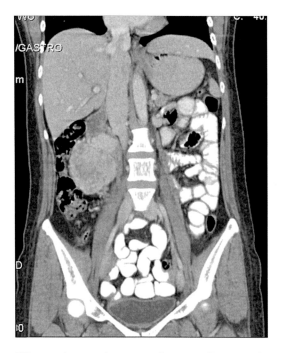

FIG. 6.3 CT scan image demonstrating a well-encapsulated, exophytic mass—typical of a GIST. In this case, the tumor is arising from the second portion of the duodenum

Less common malignancies of the stomach include gastrointestinal stromal tumors, gastric carcinoids, and gastric lymphoma. **Gastrointestinal stromal tumors (GIST)** are a type of sarcoma that can occur anywhere along the GI tract, but are most commonly found in the stomach. Unlike adenocarcinoma which arises from the gastric mucosa, GISTs are derived from the interstitial cells of Cajal, located in the submucosa. As a result, GISTs have a distinct appearance: they are typically exophytic round lesions with a smooth mucosal surface (Fig. 6.3). An endoscopic ultrasound showing that the lesion originates in the submucosa is sufficient for diagnosis. Biopsy is not necessary prior to surgery, but if performed will demonstrate **spindle cells**. Unlike gastric adenocarcinoma,

GISTs are well-encapsulated require neither extensive margins nor a lymph node dissection. However, even after complete resection, GISTs may recur locally or may present with liver or lung metastases.

The vast majority of GISTs express an activating mutation in the gene that encodes for **c-kit**, a tyrosine kinase whose constitutive activation leads to unchecked cell growth. This feature of GISTs can be targeted using the agent **imatinib**, a tyrosine kinase inhibitor. Imatinib is indicated in patients with unresectable or metastatic GISTs, and also as adjuvant therapy in patients who are at high risk for recurrence following resection. Tumor features that imply poor prognosis include size larger than 5 cm and a high mitotic rate.

Surgical Technique

The simplest type of gastrectomy is a **wedge resection**, or sleeve gastrectomy, where a portion of the greater curvature is resected without compromising the gastric lumen. This type of resection is generally reserved for benign processes or for tumor types that do not require extensive margins (e.g., GIST and gastric carcinoid). With larger wedge resections it is important to ensure that the channel of the stomach is not narrowed or occluded; some surgeons will pass a bougie from the mouth into the duodenum to ensure patency. Because the stomach is very distensible, a significant portion of the stomach can be taken in this manner without limiting normal food intake.

More extensive gastric resections include in increasing order: **distal gastrectomy**, **subtotal gastrectomy**, and **total gastrectomy** (Fig. 6.4). All these procedures begin by dividing the greater omentum between the stomach and the transverse colon in order to enter the lesser sac. Mobilization of the stomach is carried out by ligating the **short gastric arteries** by the spleen. These vessels must be divided to allow full mobilization of the proximal stomach. It is important not to place excessive traction on the stomach during this maneuver; if

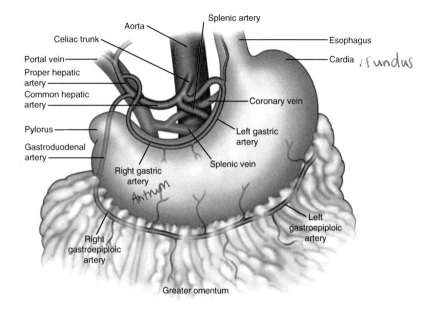

FIG. 6.4 Surgical anatomy during gastrectomy: gastroesophageal junction, cardia, antrum, pylorus, lesser curvature, greater curvature, celiac trunk, left gastric artery, splenic artery, common hepatic artery, right gastric artery, gastroduodenal artery, coronary vein, right gastroepiploic artery, left gastroepiploic artery, greater omentum, and lesser omentum

avulsed, these vessels are notorious for their ability to cause significant intraoperative hemorrhage. The **right gastric artery** is divided and the duodenum is divided approximately 1 cm past the pylorus. The proximal stomach is transected at the indicated level.

Various manners of reconstruction are available to reconnect the gastric remnant to the GI tract, each with their own pros and cons. A **Billroth I** reconstruction (**gastroduodenostomy**) directly anastomoses the stomach remnant to the duodenal stump; this requires a single anastomosis and as a result has the lowest incidence of leaks. This reconstruction is also appealing because it most closely recreates normal anatomy and physiology. However, its use is limited by the fact that the duodenum has limited mobility and cannot reach if a large segment of the stomach has been resected. Therefore only a distal gastrectomy can be reconnected in this manner.

In a **Billroth II** reconstruction (**gastrojejunostomy**), the duodenum is left blind and the gastric remnant is anastomosed to the proximal jejunum, thus creating one anastomosis and leaving a suture line at the duodenal stump. Due to its ease, this reconstruction is the most commonly used method to restore GI continuity, but is associated with a slightly higher rate of postoperative complications including a **duodenal stump leak**.

The reconstruction method after a subtotal gastrectomy is a **Roux-en-Y gastrojejunostomy**, and the correlate for total gastrectomy is a **Roux-en-Y esophagojejunostomy**. A jejunal limb of approximately 50 cm in length is created to separate the alimentary limb from the pancreaticobiliary limb. This reconstruction involves three suture lines: the duodenal stump, the gastrojejunostomy (or esophagojejunostomy), and the jejunojejunostomy, and therefore has a greater number of potential leak sites.

Complications

Anastomotic leaks, bleeding, and wound infections are possible after gastrectomy as with any GI surgery. In addition to these, there is a cluster of complications specifically related to gastric surgery known collectively as **post-gastrectomy syndromes**.

Bile esophagitis occurs from reflux of small intestinal contents up into the esophagus. Patients present with epigastric pain and burning similar to acid reflux, but the symptoms are not relieved by antacids, since the fluid is alkaline. This syndrome occurs when too small a small gastric remnant is connected directly to the jejunum (Billroth II anastomosis), allowing direct reflux of enteric contents into the esophagus. Conversion to a Roux-en-Y is curative because it separates the biliary and enteric limbs, and should be considered for patients with severe symptoms.

Afferent limb syndrome is caused by angulation or kinking of the duodenal limb of a Billroth II. As the biliary and pancreatic secretions build up, the obstructed portion of bowel becomes progressively dilated, causing abdominal pain. Ultimately, the increased pressure within this loop overcomes the point of obstruction, and leads to sudden bilious emesis, with immediate relief of pain.

Dumping syndrome describes the combined symptoms of flushing, diaphoresis, cramping, and diarrhea that occur after ingestion of a meal. Although described as one entity, dumping syndrome can be separated into two distinct processes. **Early dumping** occurs within minutes of eating, and is due to the rapid passage of food from the stomach into the small intestine; this causes a massive fluid shift into the intestinal lumen, leading to symptoms. **Late dumping** occurs a couple hours after a meal, and is due to the load of carbohydrates in the small intestine with resultant hyperinsulinemia and hypoglycemia. Both syndromes can generally be managed with dietary modifications.

Classic Case

A 52-year-old Chinese man presents with vague abdominal pain and weight loss. He states that he recently completed a course of triple therapy for *H. pylori* infection, but continues to be symptomatic. An upper endoscopy is performed which reveals a 3 cm erosion along the lesser curvature of the stomach. Biopsies from this site demonstrate poorly differentiated gastric adenocarcinoma. A CT scan does not indicate any metastatic disease. A diagnostic laparoscopy is performed, no obvious carcinomatosis is seen, and cytology from the lavage is negative for malignant cells. An endoscopic ultrasound is performed and reveals multiple enlarged lymph nodes indicating locally advanced disease. The patient undergoes a course of neoadjuvant chemotherapy. Repeat CT imaging confirms no metastases have developed, and he is scheduled for gastrectomy.

A subtotal gastrectomy with Roux-en-Y reconstruction is performed, along with a D2 lymphadenectomy. The patient has an uneventful postoperative recovery and upon discharge is instructed to eat six small meals per day. The pathology report reveals a yT3N1 tumor. He completes adjuvant chemotherapy and is enrolled in regular imaging to survey for recurrence.

OR Questions

1. What is gastric outlet obstruction?
   Gastric outlet obstruction is a phenomenon that occurs when the outflow of the stomach is blocked and the proximal stomach becomes massively dilated (Fig. 6.5). This obstruction can either be due to a distal gastric malignancy, or from chronic peptic ulcer disease where the peri-pyloric region becomes scarred and fibrosed.

2. Which vitamin deficiency can occur following total gastrectomy?
   The parietal cells of the stomach secrete intrinsic factor that binds vitamin B12 and allows its absorption in the terminal ileum. In the absence of intrinsic factor this vitamin cannot be absorbed. As a result, supplementation of B12 is necessary following total gastrectomy.

3. What are risk factors for infection with *H. pylori*?
   H. pylori is usually acquired in childhood and is found in higher rates in individuals from developing countries. The risk is especially high if a family member has been infected with H. pylori.

4. A patient with known *peptic ulcer disease* presents with a massive upper GI bleed, what is the likely cause?
   Erosion of a posterior duodenal ulcer into the gastroduodenal artery, causing brisk arterial bleeding.

5. What is Virchow's node?
   Metastases to a left supraclavicular lymph node, commonly seen in gastric or pancreatic adenocarcinoma.

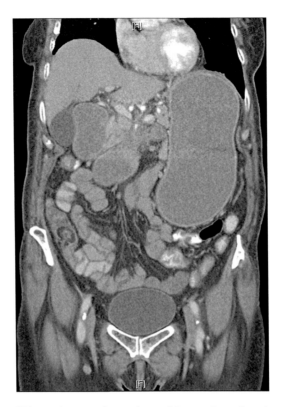

FIG. 6.5 CT scan image of a patient with gastric outlet obstruction secondary to gastric adenocarcinoma; note the massively dilated proximal stomach

6. What is linitus plastica?
   Extensive submucosal spread of gastric cancer involving the entire stomach which gives the appearance of a "leather bottle."
7. What are signet ring cells and what is their significance?
   Signet ring cells indicate a poorly differentiated tumor; this type of cancer is more often seen in young patients and unfortunately confers a dismal prognosis.

8. Two years following a distal gastrectomy for locally advanced adenocarcinoma, a patient presents to the emergency room with symptoms of small bowel obstruction. What are the two most likely etiologies of this obstruction?

In general, adhesions are the most likely cause of small bowel obstruction following prior surgery. However in a patient with a history of gastric cancer, bowel obstruction secondary to carcinomatosis must also be considered. A CT scan and/or diagnostic laparoscopy may be needed to establish the diagnosis.

Gastrectomy

Peptic ulcer disease
- Surgical emergencies: perforated ulcer, bleeding ulcer (gastroduodenal artery), gastric outlet obstruction
- Main stimuli of acid secretion by the parietal cells are eliminated with antrectomy (resection of the gastrin producing G-cells) plus vagotomy (prevents acetylcholine stimulation)
- Surgical treatment less common since widespread use of proton pump inhibitors and H.pylori treatment

Helicobacter pylori
- Infection occurs in childhood
- Infection clusters in families
- More common in developing countries
- Risk factor for both ulcers and gastric cancer
- Treatment with triple therapy to eradicate bacteria

Gastric adenocarcinoma
- Risk factors: Helicobacter pylori, Asian ethnicity, diets high in cured meats, prior partial gastrectomy
- May present as a non-healing ulcer
- Diagnosis made by upper endoscopy and biopsy
- Staging: CT scan to assess for liver metastases, diagnostic laparoscopy to rule out carcinomatosis
- Endoscopic ultrasound may be used to assess tumor depth and nodal involvement
- Consider use of neoadjuvant chemotherapy for locally advanced tumors
- Extensive submucosal tumor spread requires wide resection margins
- Need for extended lymphadenectomy is controversial, but a minimum of 16 nodes is required for complete staging

Gastro Intestinal Stromal Tumor (GIST)

- Spindle cell tumors arising from the cells of Cajal in the submucosa
- Favorable prognostic features include gastric location, size <5 cm, and low mitotic rate
- Unlike gastric adenocarcinoma, wide resection margins and lymph node dissection are not needed for GIST
- Tumors carry mutation in gene for c-kit, a tyrosine kinase receptor; Constitutive activation leads to uncontrolled cell replication
- Imitanib—tyrosine kinase inhibitor that is indicated for metastatic, unresectable, or resected but high-risk tumors

Technique

- Lesser sac is entered
- Mobilization of stomach, with ligation of short gastric vessels
- Ligation of right gastric and right gastroepiploic arteries, and left gastric artery as indicated
- Division of duodenum 1 cm past pylorus
- Resection of proximal stomach (6 cm margins needed for adenocarcinoma)
- Regional lymphadenectomy for adenocarcinoma cases
- Reconstruction of GI continuity with stapled or hand-sewn anastomosis: Billroth I gastroduodenostomy, Billroth II gastrojejunostomy, or Roux-en-Y

Peri-op orders

- Pre-incision antibiotics
- NGT per surgeon preference
- Contrast study in select cases to evaluate for leak
- Advance diet as tolerated
- Nutrition consultation for post-gastrectomy diet teaching
- Patients undergoing total gastrectomy require life-long vitamin B12 supplementation

Complications

- Anastomotic leak
- Duodenal stump leak
- B12 deficiency (if total gastrectomy)
- Bile esophagitis: reflux of alkaline jejunal contents into the esophagus causes epigastric pain and burning
- Afferent limb syndrome: intermittent obstruction due to kinking of the duodenal limb, pressure within the bowel leads to sudden bilious emesis with relief of symptoms
- Early dumping: rapid passage of food into the small intestine causes a sudden shift of fluid into the intestinal lumen, leading to pain and diarrhea
- Late dumping: rapid delivery of carbohydrates into the small intestine results in sudden insulin secretion, leading to hypoglycemia, diaphoresis, light-headedness, and tachycardia

Suggested Reading

Russell MC, Hsu C, Mansfield PF. Primary Gastric Malignancies. In: Feig BW, editor. The MD Anderson Surgical Oncology Handbook. Philadelphia. 5th ed. Lippincott Williams & Wilkins; 2012.

7
Cholecystectomy

Introduction

The gallbladder serves to store and concentrate bile until its secretion is stimulated by the ingestion of a fat-containing meal. Bile contains lecithin, bile salts, and cholesterol—an imbalance in the ratio of these components leads to the precipitation of stones, known as **cholelithiasis**. It is estimated that more than 15 % of the population has gallstones, but only a minority of these individuals will ever become symptomatic during their lifetime. Therefore, the incidental finding of cholelithiasis in an asymptomatic patient is not an indication for surgery. However, gallstones can cause several disorders that do warrant surgery.

Biliary colic describes the symptoms caused when a gallstone transiently occludes the cystic duct. This obstruction leads to distension of the gallbladder and causes intense right upper quadrant pain, accompanied by nausea and vomiting. The pain lasts for approximately 4–6 h and is self-limited, resolving when the offending stone becomes dislodged. It is important to note that in biliary colic no infection is present, and accordingly the patient will have no fever, tenderness, or leukocytosis. The treatment of biliary colic is bowel rest and intravenous hydration until the event passes, and elective cholecystectomy to prevent future attacks.

Cholecystitis occurs when the stone occluding the cystic duct remains impacted, leading to stasis and infection of the

U. Sarpel, *Surgery: An Introductory Guide*,
DOI 10.1007/978-1-4939-0903-2_7,
© Springer Science+Business Media New York 2014

bile within the gallbladder. As opposed to biliary colic, the pain of cholecystitis does not abate, and can last for days if no treatment is provided. Since infection is present, the patient will often display fever and leukocytosis. On examination, the inflamed gallbladder will cause pain on palpation of the right upper quadrant. Since the gallbladder lies under the rib cage, a special maneuver may be necessary to elicit this tenderness. A **Murphy's Sign** is performed by asking the patient to take a deep breath while the examiner is pressing into the right upper quadrant. The sign is positive when the patient has an arrest of inspiratory effort, due to the sudden pain caused by the descending gallbladder meeting the examiner's hand. The treatment of cholecystitis is bowel rest, intravenous anti-biotics, and prompt cholecystectomy. If the operation cannot be performed expeditiously, then antibiotics alone will usu-ally cause resolution of the infection and the patient can undergo surgery at a later date. However, this approach leads to a longer and more costly hospital course.

Occasionally a patient with cholecystitis is too acutely ill to undergo immediate cholecystectomy. This is unusual but may be the case in elderly, hospitalized patients with multiple comorbidities. In this circumstance, it may be more prudent to temporarily decompress the gallbladder with a **cholecys-tostomy tube** (Fig. 7.1). This minimally invasive procedure drains the infected bile, allowing the cholecystitis to resolve. However, as long as the offending stone remains impacted in the cystic duct, the cholecystostomy tube cannot be removed or else the cholecystitis will recur. Most patients can undergo cholecystectomy in a few weeks, once their underlying medical issues have been stabilized.

If a stone from the gallbladder escapes into the common bile duct, this is termed **choledocholithiasis** (Fig. 7.2). Most stones that are less than 1 cm in diameter will pass through the **Ampulla of Vater** and exit into the duodenum without incident. However, there are two potentially severe complica-tions of choledocholithiasis: cholangitis and gallstone pancre-atitis. If instead of passing smoothly though the ampulla, the stone becomes lodged and causes biliary obstruction, infection

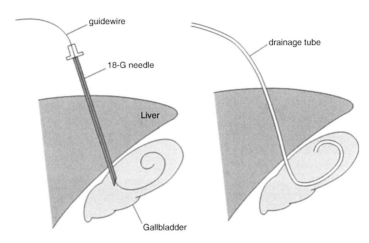

FIG. 7.1 Cholecystostomy tube placement [Reprinted from Tsuyuguchi T, Itoi T, Takada T, et al. TG13 indications and techniques for gallbladder drainage in acute cholecystitis (with videos). Journal of Hepato-Biliary-Pancreatic Sciences 2013; 20(1): 81-88. With permission from Springer Japan.]

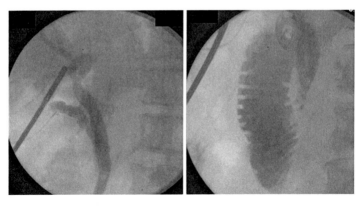

FIG. 7.2 Intraoperative cholangiogram demonstrating a stone in the common bile duct (choledocholithiasis)

of the static bile will result in **cholangitis**. Because the infected area includes the entire intrahepatic biliary tree, cholangitis rapidly progresses to bacteremia and sepsis, and can be fatal. Decompression of the biliary tree is urgently required for the treatment of cholangitis. Three different routes can be used to access the bile duct; in order of increasing invasiveness, these are endoscopic retrograde cholangiography, percutaneous transhepatic drainage, or operative common bile duct exploration. While intravenous antibiotics are also administered for cholangitis, they alone are insufficient without drainage of the biliary tree. Once the acute infection has resolved, cholecystectomy is performed to prevent future episodes.

Another serious complication of choledocholithiasis is **gallstone pancreatitis**. It is thought that the passage of a stone through the Ampulla of Vater causes irritation of the pancreatic duct with activation of pancreatic zymogens inside the pancreas. Although the stone itself passes into the duodenum, the damage has been done, and pancreatitis ensues. The treatment of gallstone pancreatitis is the same as for pancreatitis of other etiologies, and revolves around supportive care. Antibiotics are not used in uncomplicated cases of pancreatitis since the process is an inflammatory, not an infectious one. Once the acute illness has resolved, cholecystectomy is performed to remove the source of future stones. Cholangitis and gallstone pancreatitis are serious enough conditions that—unlike asymptomatic cholelithiasis—the finding of choledocholithiasis always warrants stone extraction and cholecystectomy, even in the absence of symptoms.

Occasionally other pathologies are indications for cholecystectomy. **Gallbladder cancer** is a rare malignancy that is usually asymptomatic until advanced stages. For all but the earliest stages of cancer, the gallbladder must be removed en bloc with the adjacent liver tissue and surrounding lymph nodes.

Gallstone ileus is another rare indication for cholecystectomy. This disorder is actually not an ileus, but is a mechanical small bowel obstruction caused by a gallstone that has eroded through the gallbladder wall into the adjacent duodenum, and has become lodged at the level of the ileocecal valve. Air from the bowel fills the biliary tree; as such, the presence of **pneumobilia** on imaging is pathognomonic. Surgery for gallstone ileus should be staged: the first operation should be limited to an enterotomy to remove the obstructing, the cholecystectomy and closure of the cholecysto-duodenal fistula should be performed electively once the inflammation in the region has subsided.

Surgical Technique

Laparoscopic cholecystectomy is the standard approach for removal of the gallbladder, although conversion to open surgery via a right subcostal incision may be necessary in difficult cases. After establishing pneumoperitoneum, the fundus of the gallbladder is grasped and elevated up over the liver, allowing visualization of the hilum (Fig. 7.3). The peritoneal reflection at this site is carefully incised and the fat of the gallbladder mesentery is dissected. **Calot's node** is usually encountered in this location and is mobilized off the underlying structures. The guiding principle of cholecystectomy is the definitive identification of the **cystic artery** and the **cystic duct** in order to avoid injury to the **hepatic artery** or **common bile duct**.

One method of ensuring correct anatomy is to always obtain the **critical view of safety** before ligation of any structure. In this approach, the fat in the hepatocystic triangle is dissected away until the liver bed on the opposite side can be seen with only two structures traversing the field; by definition these can only be the cystic duct and cystic artery. These two structures are then clipped and divided.

An **intraoperative cholangiogram** may be performed routinely, or as indicated to assess for the presence of choledocholithiasis or to rule out bile duct injury (Fig. 7.2). The gallbladder side of the cystic duct is clipped, and an incision is made in the downstream cystic duct. A thin catheter, introduced into the abdomen through a small stab incision, is guided into the cystic duct and clipped into place. Contrast dye is then injected

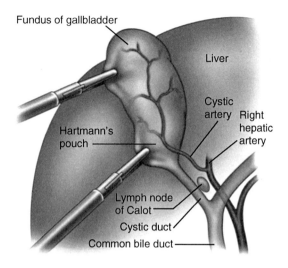

Fundus of gallbladder

Liver

Cystic
artery   Right
           hepatic
           artery

Hartmann's
pouch

Lymph node
of Calot
Cystic duct
Common bile duct

Fig. 7.3 Surgical anatomy during cholecystectomy: liver, fundus, Hartmann's pouch, Calot's node, cystic artery, right hepatic artery, cystic duct, and common bile duct

into the catheter and fluoroscopy images are taken. A normal intraoperative cholangiogram will demonstrate filling of the right and left hepatic ducts and the common bile duct with flow into the duodenum.

The gallbladder is then dissected off the liver bed using electrocautery in an upward fashion. Once freed, the gallbladder is placed into a bag and removed through the umbilical trocar site.

Complications

One potential complication after cholecystectomy is a **bile leak** from the cystic duct stump (Fig. 7.4). This can occur if the tie or clip that is used to close the cystic duct stump becomes dislodged. A cystic duct stump leak is more common in cases where significant inflammation was present and the closure of the duct was tenuous. In these cases, it is sometimes

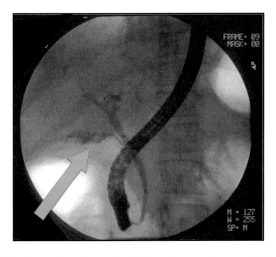

FIG. 7.4 Endoscopic retrograde cholangiogram demonstrating a bile leak from the cystic duct stump (*arrow*). [Modified from Ponsky JL. Endoluminal surgery: past, present and future. Surgical Endoscopy And Other Interventional Techniques 2006; 20(2): S500-S502. With permission from Springer Verlag.]

prudent to leave a surgical drain near the cystic duct stump in anticipation of a bile leak. The leak is self-limited in the majority of cases, and simple drainage is sufficient to temporize the situation until the leak seals off.

Although it occurs in less than 1 % of cases, the most dreaded complication of cholecystectomy is **injury to the common bile duct**. Normally, the common bile duct is not dissected out in the course of a routine cholecystectomy. However, if the surgeon becomes disoriented, or if the operation is difficult due to inflammation, then inadvertent injury to the common bile duct can occur. Most injuries to the duct are not recognized at the time of surgery. If there has been a laceration or transection of the common bile duct, bile will leak freely into the peritoneal cavity. Bile is extremely irritating to the tissues; patients will present with postoperative abdominal pain and imaging will demonstrate fluid in the abdominal cavity. If instead the common bile duct has been inadvertently ligated, the patient will present with worsening

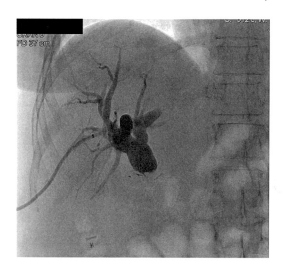

FIG. 7.5 Percutaneous transhepatic cholangiogram demonstrating an iatrogenic injury of the common bile duct caused during laparoscopic cholecystectomy. The images show complete occlusion of the common bile duct by surgical clips; note the proximal intrahepatic biliary dilatation

jaundice, and imaging will demonstrate biliary dilatation proximal to the obstruction (Fig. 7.5). Treatment of a common bile duct injury almost always requires restoration of biliary-enteric continuity with a **hepaticojejunostomy**.

Classic Case

A 45-year-old woman presents to the emergency room complaining of right upper quadrant pain for 2 days. She had similar attacks of pain when she was pregnant, but none of this duration. She reports fevers at home, and complains of nausea with emesis. Her vital signs are normal except a fever to 39 °C. Her abdominal exam is non-tender, but she does have a positive **Murphy's sign**. Lab values demonstrate a leukocytosis of $14.5 \times 10^3/\mu L$, and normal liver function tests. An ultrasound demonstrates a thickened gallbladder wall, gallstones, and pericholecystic fluid. She is admitted, given intravenous antibiotics, and scheduled for a laparoscopic cholecystectomy.

At surgery, there is an intense inflammatory response making dissection difficult and the decision is made to convert to a subcostal incision. The anatomy is clarified allowing the cystic duct and cystic artery to be identified and safely ligated. The gallbladder is dissected off the liver bed, and passed off the field. A cholangiogram demonstrates normal anatomy, no evidence of biliary injury, and no choledocholithiasis. A drain is placed near the cystic duct stump. She has an uneventful recovery, the drain output remains nonbilious, and is removed prior to her discharge home.

OR Questions

1. Which is a better test to look for gallstones, CT or ultrasonography?
   Ultrasonography. CT is inferior for several reasons. First, approximately 1/3rd of gallstones are not dense enough to be visible on CT. In addition, CT is costly and exposes the patient to unnecessary radiation and intravenous contrast. Ultrasound is cheap, fast, harmless, and provides excellent visualization of gallstones.
2. What are the sonographic findings of biliary colic?
   Cholelithiasis only.
3. What are the sonographic findings of cholecystitis?
   Cholelithiasis, gallbladder wall thickening, and pericholecystic fluid.
4. One week after a routine laparoscopic cholecystectomy, a patient presents to the office with jaundice. What is the diagnosis?
   Iatrogenic ligation of the common bile duct, until proven otherwise.
5. What is **Charcot's triad** and what does its presence indicate?
   Fever, jaundice, and right upper quadrant pain. The presence of Charcot's triad is pathognomonic of cholangitis.

6. What is **Reynaud's pentad** and what does it indicate?
   Charcot's triad, plus hypotension and altered mental status. The presence of Reynaud's Pentad indicates that the patient's cholangitis has progressed to septic shock.

7. How soon should cholecystectomy be performed following gallstone pancreatitis?
   As soon as the patient's pancreatitis has resolved. The recurrence rate of gallstone pancreatitis is quite high, and patients should not be discharged home prior to cholecystectomy.

Cholecystectomy

Cholelithiasis
- The majority of patients with gallstones will remain asymptomatic and surgery is not indicated
- Biliary colic: steady right upper quadrant pain lasting for a few hours, associated with nausea and vomiting
- Biliary colic occurs when a gallstone transiently obstructs the cystic duct
- Ultrasound is normal except for the presence of gallstones

Gallstone ileus
- Small bowel obstruction caused by the erosion of a gallstone through the gallbladder wall directly into the duodenum
- The stone causes obstruction at the level of the ileocecal valve, the narrowest point in the bowel
- Pneumobilia is pathognomonic
- Staged surgery: first enterotomy to remove stone is performed, cholecystectomy and closure of the cholecysto-duodenal fistula is performed electively after recovery

Cholecystitis
- Occurs when a gallstone obstructs the cystic duct, leading to stasis and infection of the bile in the gall bladder
- Pain is constant and persists for hours to days
- Fever, tenderness, and leukocytosis are typically present
- Murphy's sign: arrest of inspiratory effort during pressure on the right upper quadrant
- Ultrasonography shows gallstones, thickened gallbladder wall, and pericholecystic fluid
- Treatment is intravenous antibiotics and cholecystectomy

Gallstone pancreatitis
- Passage of gallstone through the common channel of bile duct and pancreatic duct leads to irritation of pancreas and activation of zymogens
- Cholecystectomy is indicated after recovery to prevent future episodes

Ascending cholangitis
- Obstruction of the common bile duct with infection
- Can be rapidly life-threatening
- Charcot's triad: abdominal pain, jaundice, and fever
- Reynaud's pentad: the triad plus hypotension and mental status changes, indicating the onset of septic shock
- Treatment involves antibiotics and emergent decompression of the duct by endoscopic or transhepatic approach
- Cholecystectomy is indicated after recovery to prevent future episodes

Gallbladder cancer
- Rare tumor
- Usually asymptomatic until later stages
- May be found incidentally on cholecystectomy
- Depending on the stage, the gallbladder must be removed en bloc with the adjacent liver tissue and surrounding lymph nodes

Imaging
- Ultrasound is the preferred imaging test, since is it inexpensive, safe, and 1/3rd of gallstones are not visible on CT scan
- The common bile duct cannot be seen on ultrasound due to gas in the overlying duodenum
- Cholescintigraphy can be used if the diagnosis is uncertain; failure of the gallbladder to fill confirms obstruction of the cystic duct

Intraoperative cholangiography
- The cystic duct stump is cannulated and injected with contrast to allow visualization of the biliary tree
- Cholangiography may be performed routinely on all patients, or selectively as indicated by:
- Preoperative indications: history of gallstone pancreatitis or cholangitis, biliary dilatation on imaging, hx of elevated bilirubin
- Intraoperative indications: unclear anatomy, concern for bile duct injury

Technique: Laparoscopic cholecystectomy
- The fundus is grasped and elevated
- Dissection of Calot's triangle
- Identification of cystic duct
- Consider cholangiography
- Ligation of cystic duct
- Identification and ligation of cystic artery
- Dissection of gallbladder off liver bed
- Removal of specimen and closure of trocar sites
- Open cholecystectomy is indicated for difficult dissections

Peri-op orders
- Pre-incision antibiotics
- Consider drain placement for cases with high potential for bile leak
- Advance diet as tolerated
- Uncomplicated laparoscopic cases may be discharged home the same day

Complications
- Cystic duct stump bile leak: usually self-limited, or resolves with endoscopic sphincterotomy
- Common bile duct injury: usually requires hepaticojejunostomy
- Retained common duct stones: requires endoscopic sphincterotomy and stone extraction

Suggested Reading

Sarpel U, Pachter HL. Cholecystitis, cholangitis, and jaundice. In: Britt LD, Peitzman AB, Barie PS, Jurkovich GJ, editors. Acute care surgery. 1st ed. Philadelphia: Lippincott Williams & Wilkins; 2012.

8

Hepatectomy

Introduction

Although historically one of the later fields to develop, liver surgery is now widely performed for a variety of benign and malignant disorders. Safe liver resection has become possible due to a better understanding of hepatic anatomy, the development of more effective hemostatic techniques, and improved patient selection.

One of the most intriguing aspects of the liver is its remarkable capacity to regenerate lost tissue. Starting within hours after resection, the remaining liver cells begin to undergo division; within 1 month of surgery, the liver remnant will have regenerated back to its preoperative volume. During this period of regeneration, a patient undergoing liver resection must retain enough functional parenchyma to support vital functions. In an individual with a normal liver, up to 80 % of the liver parenchyma can be resected, without risk of postoperative liver failure. By contrast, the cirrhotic liver is markedly limited in its ability to regenerate. Depending on the degree of dysfunction, cirrhotic patients may not tolerate even a minor hepatectomy. Therefore, careful patient selection is critical to the practice of safe liver surgery.

Hepatic **metastasectomy** is one of the most common indications for liver surgery. While not indicated for all cancers, resection of liver metastases can prolong survival in certain tumor types. For example, while patients with metastatic

U. Sarpel, *Surgery: An Introductory Guide*,
DOI 10.1007/978-1-4939-0903-2_8,

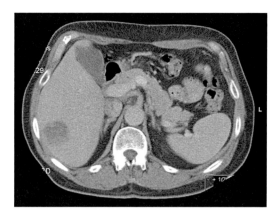

FIG. 8.1 Axial CT scan image of a patient with a single liver metastasis of colorectal origin

pancreatic cancer do not benefit from resection of liver metastases, resection of **colorectal liver metastases** can significantly improve survival in appropriately selected patients (Fig. 8.1). These differences are partially due to differences in tumor aggressiveness, and also to the efficacy of available systemic chemotherapy for that tumor type.

In patients with metastatic colorectal cancer, several clinical features have been shown to identify the best candidates for hepatectomy. In general, patients who are most likely to benefit from resection of colorectal liver metastases are those who display less aggressive tumor biology, as evidenced by a long disease-free interval, no extrahepatic metastases, low carcinoembryonic antigen (CEA) levels, lack of lymph node metastases, and fewer and smaller liver lesions. Hepatic metastasectomy has also shown to be of survival benefit to select patients with metastases from other cancers such as a pancreatic endocrine tumor, carcinoid tumor, gastrointestinal stromal tumor, and sarcoma. Patients with liver metastases from other primaries may be advised to undergo hepatectomy on a case-by-case basis.

The liver can also develop primary tumors, including **hepatocellular carcinoma** (HCC), which arises from hepatocytes,

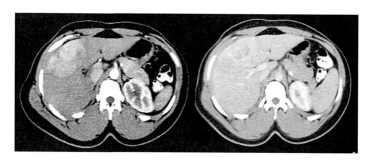

FIG. 8.2 Arterial and venous phase images of a patient with a hepatocellular carcinoma; note the typical pattern of enhancement and washout

and **cholangiocarcinoma**, which arises from the biliary cells of the liver. Of these, HCC is much more common, with the majority of cases developing in the setting of preexisting **cirrhosis** (Fig. 8.2). A wide variety of diseases can lead to cirrhosis of the liver including **hepatitis B**, **hepatitis C**, **alcoholic liver disease**, **nonalcoholic fatty liver disease**, alpha-1 antitrypsin deficiency, hemochromatosis, etc. It is important to recognize that all patients with cirrhosis are at risk for the subsequent development of hepatocellular carcinoma, regardless of the underlying etiology. In addition, hepatitis B is unique in its ability to cause HCC even in the absence of cirrhosis. In the USA, hepatitis C and alcoholic cirrhosis are the most common causes of HCC. By contrast, in much of East Asia and sub-Saharan Africa, infection with hepatitis B is by far the most frequent etiology. The recent development of a vaccine for hepatitis B has started to decrease the incidence of HCC in some countries; however limited distribution in developing countries remains a significant barrier.

HCC does not cause symptoms until advanced stages; therefore patients who are at high-risk must undergo routine imaging screening in order to detect HCC at a treatable stage. The only curative options for HCC are **hepatectomy** or **liver transplantation**. Thermal **ablation** of the tumor may be equally effective as surgery in patients with a single small

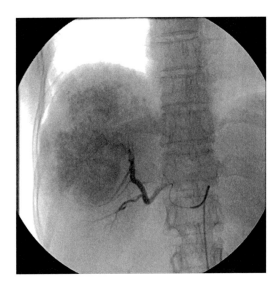

Fɪɢ. 8.3 Chemoembolization of a large hepatocellular carcinoma in the right hepatic lobe

lesion (e.g., <2 cm). If a patient is not a candidate for any of these therapies, less effective alternatives such as **emboliza-tion** may be considered (Fig. 8.3). HCC is predominantly fed by branches of the hepatic artery, therefore selective emboli-zation of the hepatic artery creates tumor necrosis, while the surrounding normal liver parenchyma is preserved by blood from the portal vein. In patients with metastatic HCC, **sorafenib** is an oral agent that has been shown to prolong survival.

Liver surgery is also occasionally performed for benign lesions. Hepatic hemangiomas and liver cysts are two com-mon benign entities that only rarely require intervention. However, if sufficiently large, these lesions can cause symp-tomatic gastric compression, or painful stretching of the liver capsule, which may require surgery for relief (Fig. 8.4). **Hepatic adenoma** is a benign tumor of the liver that can undergo malignant degeneration or spontaneous hemor-rhage, particularly if it exceeds 5 cm in size. This tumor is

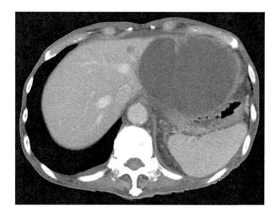

Fɪɢ. 8.4 CT image of a patient with a large hepatic cyst; note the marked gastric compression caused by the mass and the patient's lack of subcutaneous fat, consistent with limited food intake

stimulated by the presence of estrogen, and therefore resection is generally recommended in premenopausal women if the lesion is approaching this size. An additional indication for hepatic resection is in those patients who wish to donate a portion of their liver for liver transplantation.

Surgical Technique

Safe liver surgery is predicated on a solid understanding of the segmental anatomy of the liver and knowledge of the vascular inflow and outflow (Fig. 8.5). The type of incision used for liver surgery depends on the location of the lesion, the extent of the planned resection, and surgeon preference. Commonly used incisions are a modified subcostal incision, a chevron incision with extension toward the xiphoid, and the standard midline incision. Laparoscopic liver resection is becoming increasingly performed at specialized centers, however is generally limited to easily accessible lesions in the periphery of the liver.

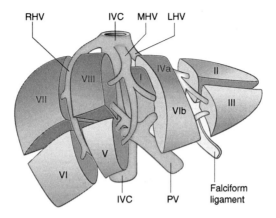

FIG. 8.5 Segmental anatomy of the liver. [Reprinted from Randone
B, Matteotti R, Gayet B. Liver—Anatomical Liver Resections. In:
Matteotti R, Ashley SW (eds). Minimally Invasice Surgical Oncology:
State-of-the-Art Cancer Management. Heidelberg, Germany:
Springer Verlag; 2011:273-296 with permission from Springer Verlag]

Once access to the abdomen has been established, the
liver must be mobilized from its attachments (Fig. 8.6). The
gallbladder lies along the line that delineates the right and
left lobes of the liver. As a result, a cholecystectomy must be
performed as a part of any right or left hepatectomy. Next, a
dissection of the **porta hepatis** is performed to identify the
hepatic artery, common bile duct, and portal vein. The right
or left branches of these structures are carefully ligated and
divided, according to the side to be resected. In a right hepatectomy for example, the right hepatic artery is ligated and
divided, followed by the right branch of the portal vein. This
leads to ischemic demarcation of the right lobe of the liver.
Next the right bile duct is divided. Once this is complete, the
outflow vessels of the liver are identified. Small venous
branches from the liver to the inferior vena cava, known as
the **short hepatic veins**, are carefully divided. Finally, the right
hepatic vein is dissected out, ligated, and transected.

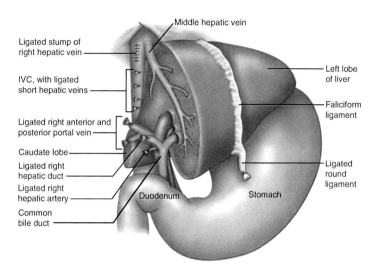

Fig. 8.6 Surgical anatomy during hepatectomy: diaphragm, inferior vena cava, right hepatic vein, middle hepatic vein, left hepatic vein, short hepatic veins, right hepatic lobe, left hepatic lobe, caudate lobe, falciform ligament, round ligament, portal vein, hepatic duct, hepatic artery, hepatoduodenal ligament, and duodenum

Once this preparation is complete, the parenchymal transection can be performed. The technique used for transection varies by surgeon, and may include the use of staplers or clips to ligate vascular and biliary branches. A **Pringle maneuver** is often employed during surgery to decrease blood loss: a clamp is placed across the hepatic artery and portal vein, thereby occluding vascular inflow. The liver is ischemic during the Pringle maneuver, therefore clamp times should be kept to a minimum. Once transection is complete, hemostasis of the cut surface of the liver is typically obtained with a combination of direct pressure, cautery, and application of prothrombotic agents.

Smaller wedge resections of the liver can be performed without extensive dissection. Depending on the location and depth, the tumor can be simply wedged out with a surrounding

margin of normal liver. Precoagulation of the liver parenchyma around the lesion is sometimes employed to facilitate
hemostatic resection.

Complications

The liver is a richly vascular organ, and massive **hemorrhage**
is a potential complication of hepatic surgery. Bleeding can
occur from laceration of any of the major vessels including
the hepatic artery, portal vein, hepatic veins, or inferior vena
cava. A clear understanding of hepatic anatomy is crucial to
avoid inadvertent injury to these structures. Additionally,
hemorrhage can occur as a result of persistent oozing from
the cut parenchymal surface. Various techniques, topical
agents, and direct manual pressure can be used to achieve
hemostasis of the liver surface. This potential for bleeding is
further complicated by the fact that liver surgery is often
performed on cirrhotic patients with some degree of preexisting coagulopathy. For these reasons, close postoperative
monitoring of hemodynamics is essential in patients undergoing hepatectomy.

Prevention of a **biliary leak** is another important aspect
of liver surgery. A bile leak can occur from damage to, or
incomplete ligation of a major branch of the biliary tree.
More commonly, however, bile leaks are from the small
radicals along the cut surface of the liver. A drain placed
along the liver remnant can be used to collect any potential
leaking fluid. Fortunately, the vast majority of bile leaks
will seal themselves off without need for further
intervention.

Postoperative **liver failure** should be rare with appropriate
patient selection. As described earlier, prior to performing a
liver resection, the surgeon must be certain that the remaining
parenchyma is of sufficient volume to support vital functions.
In patients with a borderline status, pre-operative **portal vein
embolization** can be performed. For this procedure, the

interventional radiologists use foam, coils, or embolic beads to occlude the portal vein to the lobe to be resected. This induces hypertrophy of the contralateral side, allowing a greater amount of liver remnant to support liver functions following resection.

In patients who undergo liver resection but are left with an inadequate volume of liver, signs of hepatic insufficiency such as jaundice, encephalopathy, and ascites will manifest in the days following surgery. Dialysis-like machines to sustain liver function are under development, but currently there is little more than supportive care that can be offered to these patients. This once again underscores the need for careful pre-operative evaluation of patients for liver resection.

Classic Case

A 57-year-old man with hepatitis C and cirrhosis presents with a complaint of abdominal pain. He has not seen a physician for several years and has not participated in the recommended screening for liver cancer. A CT scan is obtained which demonstrates a 4 cm lesion within the right lobe of the liver. During the arterial phase of the scan the lesion is brighter than the surrounding liver, and washes out on the venous phase, diagnostic of a hepatocellular carcinoma. His laboratory results indicate Child's A cirrhosis, and there is no evidence of portal hypertension. His AFP is 350 ng/mL. The patient undergoes right portal vein embolization, and 4 weeks later a repeat CT scan confirms significant hypertrophy of the left lobe. A right hepatic lobectomy is then performed utilizing a 15-min Pringle maneuver. Postoperatively, the patient has transient liver insufficiency, as evidenced by mild elevations in his INR and bilirubin. These values normalize over the next few days and he is ultimately discharged home.

OR Questions

1. Why is the liver the most common site of metastasis for GI organs?
   All venous blood returning from the GI tract enters the portal vein, and must first pass through the liver to enter the systemic circulation.
2. In a patient with no underlying liver disease, what is the most likely etiology of a liver tumor?
   Metastatic colorectal cancer.
3. In a patient with cirrhosis, what is the most likely etiology of a liver tumor?
   Hepatocellular carcinoma.
4. What features of cirrhosis are evident on CT or MRI imaging?
   Nodular liver surface, ascites, varices, splenomegaly, cavernous transformation of the portal vein.
5. A young woman is found to have a 3 cm hepatic adenoma on imaging. What medication should you discontinue?
   Since hepatic adenomas are stimulated by the presence of estrogen, the patient should discontinue taking any oral contraceptives.
6. What tumor markers are useful in determining the etiology of a liver lesion?
   Carcinoembryonic antigen (CEA)=metastatic colorectal cancer, alfa fetoprotein (AFP)=hepatocellular carcinoma, CA 19-9=cholangiocarcinoma or metastatic pancreatic adenocarcinoma.

Hepatectomy

Hepatocellular carcinoma
- Primary neoplasm of liver
- Occurs as a result of cirrhosis (from any etiology), or chronic hepatitis B infection without cirrhosis
- Routine screening with q6 month liver ultrasound is recommended for early detection
- Resection or transplantation are potentially curative modalities, if patient is a candidate
- Ablation is effective only for small (<2 cm) tumors
- Hepatic artery embolization slows tumor progression, but is not curative
- Sorafenib has been shown to prolong survival in patients with metastases or advanced disease

Metastasectomy
- Liver is the first site of metastases for all GI tumors due to portal venous drainage of the gut
- Resection can prolong survival in select patients, e.g. colorectal metastases
- Best candidates are those with a long disease-free interval and evidence of favorable tumor biology

Benign lesions
- Adenoma: potential for both malignant transformation and rupture, especially when >5 cm, discontinue oral contraceptives, since tumor is stimulated by hormones
- Focal nodular hyperplasia: no potential for malignant transformation, resection not indicated
- Simple cyst, Hemangioma: intervention only rarely indicated in cases of gastric compression, or painful capsular stretch

Hepatic reserve
- Can resect up to 80% of liver parenchyma in patients with no underlying liver disease
- Patients with Child-Pugh A cirrhosis can tolerate only minor resections
- Patients with more advanced cirrhosis cannot tolerate any intervention
- Platelet counts <100,000 indicate portal hypertension and are a generally contraindication for resection

Technique
- Mobilization of liver
- Ligation of short hepatic veins to the IVC
- Dissection of the porta hepatis with ligation of the hepatic artery, portal vein, and bile duct to the side to be resected
- Ligation of the hepatic vein draining the side to be resected
- Pringle maneuver
- Parenchymal transection
- Hemostasis and biliostasis

Pre-operative portal vein embolization
- In patients with borderline liver function, pre-resection hypertrophy of the contralateral side can be induced by embolization of the portal vein
- Hypertrophy of the contralateral liver is complete in approximately 4-6 weeks

Peri-op orders
- Pre-incision antibiotics
- Clear liquid diet, advance as tolerated
- Monitor for signs of liver failure
- Monitor output and quality of drain fluid

Complications
- Hemorrhage
- Bile leak
- Hepatic insufficiency

Suggested Readings

Chapman WC, Alseidi AA, Hiatt JR, Nauta RJ, Stone MD. Liver. In: Lawrence PF, editor. Essentials of general surgery. 5th ed. Philadelphia: Lippincott Williams & Wilkins; 2013.

Takayama T, Makuuchi M. Liver resection of primary tumors: hepatocellular carcinoma, cholangiocarcinoma, and gallbladder cancer. In: Clavien PA, editor. Malignant liver tumors: current and emerging therapies. 3rd ed. West Sussex: John Wiley & Sons; 2010.

9
Pancreatectomy

Introduction

The pancreas is the site of several potential pathologies and the decision on whether or not to perform pancreatectomy is dependent upon on the lesion's etiology and malignant potential. Solid lesions are the most straightforward because any solid tumor of the pancreas can be assumed to be malignant (or carry malignant potential) and should be resected if feasible. The two most common solid lesions of the pancreas are pancreatic adenocarcinoma and the pancreatic endocrine tumors. The evaluation of cystic lesions is more complex, since some can be treated with observation alone, but others have malignant potential and should be resected. Each of these etiologies is described in further detail below.

Pancreatic adenocarcinoma is the most common solid lesion of the pancreas. This cancer is known for its poor prognosis, which stems from the fact that the tumor is not usually diagnosed until advanced stages, and that current chemotherapeutic regimens are largely ineffective. When a pancreatic adenocarcinoma arises in the body or tail of the pancreas, the lesion has room to grow locally without impinging on nearby structures. Patients do not typically develop symptoms until the tumor has extended posteriorly and invaded the celiac plexus of nerves, which causes back pain. By this point, most patients have already developed liver metastases

U. Sarpel, *Surgery: An Introductory Guide*,
DOI 10.1007/978-1-4939-0903-2_9,
© Springer Science+Business Media New York 2014

and are no longer candidates for pancreatic resection. By contrast, a lesion that arises in the head of the pancreas will tend to present at an earlier stage because the tumor will obstruct the common bile duct, producing jaundice at an earlier stage.

In the absence of metastases, resectability of a pancreatic cancer is determined by whether or not the tumor involves the major blood vessels that course through the region. The superior mesenteric artery, superior mesenteric vein, and celiac trunk must all be patent and free of tumoral invasion. Certain tumors that involve only a short segment of the superior mesenteric vein can still be resected along with a vein resection. In borderline resectable cases, neoadjuvant chemotherapy can be considered, with the hopes of producing tumor shrinkage. Ultimately, even among the minority who are surgical candidates, most patients will be found to have nodal metastases upon resection, which portends a poor prognosis.

Pancreatic endocrine tumors comprise a group of tumors that are characterized by classic symptoms sets that result from hormone production. For example, **insulinoma** is a tumor that—as the name suggests—produces insulin. The high levels of circulating insulin cause what is known as **Whipple's triad**: a patient has episodes of confusion and altered mental status, corresponding with documented hypoglycemia, and these symptoms are relieved upon administration of glucose. **Gastrinomas**, with their high circulating levels of gastrin, produce fulminant peptic ulcer disease, known as **Zollinger-Ellison syndrome**. Other, more rare endocrine tumors of the pancreas include VIPoma, somatostatinoma, and glucagonoma—each with their own classic symptoms. Nonfunctioning tumors are actually the most common type of endocrine tumors. These tumors are clinically silent, and are thus either found incidentally, or are discovered when the tumor's mass effect ultimately causes symptoms (Fig. 9.1). Unlike pancreatic adenocarcinomas, endocrine tumors of the pancreas are less aggressive and patients have significantly longer survival—even with metastatic disease.

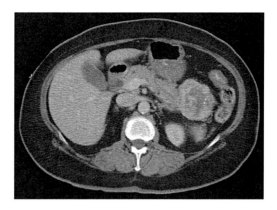

FIG. 9.1 CT scan image of a patient with a large tumor in the tail of the pancreas; at resection this was found to be a nonfunctioning pancreatic endocrine tumor

The differential diagnosis of **pancreatic cysts** includes the pseudocyst, serous cystic neoplasm, mucinous cystic neoplasm, and intraductal papillary mucinous neoplasm. The management of cystic lesions is more nuanced than solid lesions, because some are clearly benign, while others harbor malignant potential. **Pseudocysts** are the remnants of an attack of pancreatitis, and are never premalignant. These lesions usually resolve with time, although surgical intervention can be required if they persist or cause symptoms such as gastric compression. A **serous cystic neoplasm** is also a benign lesion that only rarely requires an operation. By contrast, both **mucinous cystic neoplasms** (MCN) and **intraductal papillary mucinous neoplasms** (IPMN) harbor malignant potential and should be resected, although centers differ in their specific criteria for intervention. The diagnosis of an MCN or IPMN is made by a combination of typical imaging characteristics and analysis of the cyst fluid obtained by endoscopic ultrasound guided aspiration.

Another indication for pancreatic surgery can be the sequela of **chronic pancreatitis**. The repeated bouts of inflammation can lead to scarring and strictures of the pancreatic duct. Over time, this leads to obstruction of the duct, causing postprandial pain and weight loss. In addition, the pancreatic atrophy and calcifications seen in chronic pancreatitis can obscure imaging, and make it difficult to rule out a malignant stricture. As a result, resection of the head of the pancreas is sometimes indicated.

Finally, tumors of the duodenum often require pancreatectomy due to the anatomical attachments between the duodenal sweep and the head of the pancreas. Duodenal tumors that lie in close proximity to the ampulla usually require a Whipple procedure for resection. In these cases, the pancreatectomy is just the means for performing a duodenectomy.

Surgical Technique

Different types of pancreatectomy, include a pancreaticoduodenectomy, distal pancreatectomy, total pancreatectomy, central pancreatectomy, or simple tumor enucleation, and are selected depending on the clinical case. Either a vertical midline or a chevron incision can be used depending on body habitus and surgeon preference. If a resection is being performed for pancreatic cancer, it is recommended to begin the operation with a diagnostic laparoscopy. Pancreatic adenocarcinoma is an aggressive tumor, and unexpected liver metastases or carcinomatosis are found not infrequently. Beginning with a laparoscopy spares the patient the pain and morbidity of a full incision if such metastases are discovered.

A **Whipple procedure** is the eponym for a **pancreaticoduodenectomy**, which involves the removal of the head of the pancreas, the distal bile duct, and the duodenum (Fig. 9.2). The operation begins with a **Kocher maneuver**, which is the mobilization of the duodenum and head of the pancreas from its retroperitoneal attachments. Next, the middle colic vein is followed to the **superior mesenteric vein**, which is assessed to confirm resectability. In order resect the tumor, the surgeon must be able to create a tunnel between the pancreatic neck and the underlying vein.

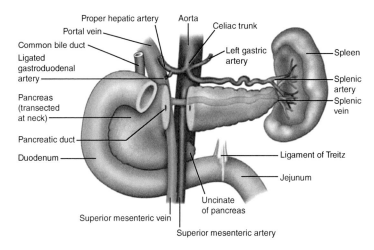

FIG. 9.2 Surgical anatomy during pancreatectomy: common bile duct, celiac trunk, splenic artery, gastroduodenal artery, hepatic artery, splenic vein, portal vein, superior mesenteric vein, superior mesenteric artery, uncinate, pancreatic duct, duodenum, ligament of Treitz

Next, a cholecystectomy and hilar dissection is performed. The common bile duct is divided just above the cystic duct junction. The gastroduodenal artery is then ligated and divided, which reveals the portal vein beneath. This exposure allows the completion of the tunnel along the superior mesenteric vein and portal vein junction. The distal stomach and proximal jejunum are transected, and finally the pancreas is transected at its neck, just above the tunnel. The uncinate process of the pancreas is carefully dissected off the superior mesenteric vein and artery, thus freeing the specimen. Reconstruction following a Whipple involves three anastomoses: a hepaticojejunostomy, pancreaticojejunostomy, and gastrojejunostomy. A pylorus-preserving Whipple utilizes a duodenojejunostomy as a variant (Fig. 9.3).

A **distal pancreatectomy** is generally a technically simpler operation since no bowel anastomoses are required, and

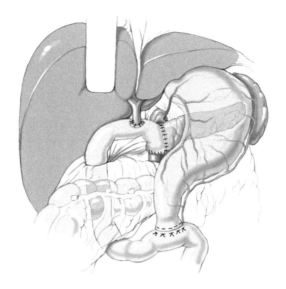

FIG. 9.3 Postoperative anatomy after pylorus-preserving pancreati-coduodenectomy. [Reprinted from Mantke R, Schulz H-U, Lippert H. Basic Chapter. In: Mantke R, Lippert H, Büchler MW, Sarr MG (eds). International Practices in Pancreatic Surgery. Heidelberg, Germany: Springer Verlag; 2013:157-163, with permission from Springer Verlag]

both laparoscopic and open versions are commonly performed. A splenectomy is typically included with a distal pancreatectomy, particularly if the tumor is invading the splenic vein or is in close proximity to the splenic hilum. Once access to the abdomen is obtained, the lesser sac is entered and the stomach is reflected upwards to expose the pancreas beneath. The peritoneum overlying the upper and lower borders of the pancreas is divided, allowing mobilization of the gland. The splenic artery and vein are ligated and divided at the level of the intended transection, often using a vascular stapler. The pancreas is then divided with a stapling device, which seals the pancreatic duct. The distal pancreas and spleen are then freed from the remaining attachments.

Complications

At high-volume centers, pancreatic resection can be performed safely with low morbidity and mortality rates. However, even in the best of hands, certain complications can occur. A **pancreatic leak** is the most serious complication of any pancreatic procedure. Of the three anastomoses during a Whipple, the pancreaticojejunostomy is the most prone to leakage. This is due to the fact that a normal pancreas is soft and sutures can easily pull through the tissue. Similarly, in a distal pancreatectomy, the sutures or staples along the stump of the pancreatic parenchyma can tear, allowing leakage of pancreatic juice from the duct (Fig. 9.4).

The first sign of a pancreatic leak is usually a fever or rise in white blood cell count a few days into the postoperative period. Occasionally the patient will be completely asymptomatic, but the drain output will become thick and greyish. The presence of a leak can be confirmed by sending the drain

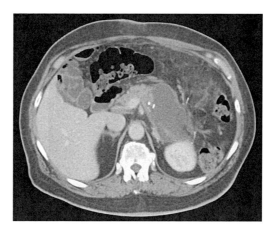

Fig. 9.4 CT scan demonstrating a leak from the tail of the pancreas following distal pancreatectomy; note the fluid collection and surrounding edema and fat stranding

output for an amylase level. The vast majority of patients with a pancreatic leak can be managed non-operatively. The key is to ensure that the leak is contained and adequately drained. A CT scan is obtained to assess the size and location of the fluid collection, and additional drains are placed as needed by interventional radiology. Drainage is usually sufficient to allow the pancreatic duct to seal off. The drain is left in place until the patient is clinically improved and the drain output has diminished.

Intraoperative hemorrhage is a potential complication of pancreatic surgery due to the close proximity of the organ to several major blood vessels. Experience and good technique are essential to avoid major blood loss. Postoperative hemorrhage should raise the suspicion of an underlying pancreatic leak. The enzyme-rich fluid that leaks from the pancreatic duct can erode into one of the many nearby vessels causing massive bleeding. Embolization of the bleeding site in interventional radiology is the most effective treatment of this complication.

Classic Case

A 68-year-old woman presents to her doctor after a colleague has pointed out that her eyes seem yellow. She is asymptomatic other than mild fatigue and reports recent weight loss of about 10 lbs. Blood work reveals a direct bilirubin level of 15 mg/dL and a CA 19-9 level of 108 U/mL. An ultrasound demonstrates significant intra- and extrahepatic biliary dilatation and a dilated gallbladder without stones. She undergoes a CT scan that reveals a 2 cm tumor in the head of the pancreas without encroachment upon the major vessels. No evidence of metastases is seen.

She undergoes a diagnostic laparoscopy that does not reveal any carcinomatosis, followed by a pancreaticoduodenectomy. Her initial recovery is uneventful, but on the 5th postoperative day, the output from her surgical drain becomes a greyish, murky fluid. A sample of the fluid reveals an amylase of 3,000 U/L. A CT scan is obtained which demonstrates a collection posterior to the pancreas, with the drain in adequate position. The patient remains asymptomatic and clinically stable. Her diet is slowly advanced and she is discharged home on the 8th postoperative day with the drain in place. When she is seen a week later in the office, the drain output is minimal, and the drain is removed without incident. The pathology report reveals pancreatic adenocarcinoma with lymphatic metastases, and she is referred to medical oncology for evaluation for adjuvant chemo therapy.

OR Questions

1. A patient presents with the sudden onset of jaundice, accompanied by fever and abdominal pain. What is the likely etiology?
   These symptoms are most likely due to biliary obstruction by a stone in the common bile duct. By contrast, a pancreatic tumor causes slow, insidious biliary obstruction in the absence of other symptoms.
2. What tumor marker is associated with pancreatic adenocarcinoma?
   CA 19-9.
3. What is Courvoisier's sign, and what diagnosis does it suggest?
   A palpable, distended, but non-tender gallbladder. This passive distention of the gallbladder dilation suggests a slow, progressive downstream biliary obstruction, classically a pancreatic cancer.
4. In a patient with an unresectable tumor in the head of the pancreas, how should the jaundice be treated?
   Endoscopic retrograde cholangiography with biliary stenting is a minimally invasive way to restore drainage of bile and allow resolution of jaundice.
5. A patient presents with loss of consciousness and is found to have a glucose level of 27 mg/dL. What blood test will differentiate between an insulinoma and self-administration of exogenous insulin?

Insulin is naturally produced when C-peptide is cleaved off proinsulin. However, injectable insulin does not contain C-peptide. Therefore, a C-peptide level will be low if the hypoglycemia is due to an exogenous insulin overdose.

6. An 87-year-old man with multiple comorbidities is found to have a small IPMN on a CT obtained for other reasons. What is the recommended management?

   IPMN is a lesion with the potential to undergo malignant transformation, and resection is indicated in certain cases to prevent this occurrence. However in this elderly patient with a limited life span who is high-risk for surgery, observation alone is sufficient.

7. Would the fluid within a pseudocyst contain low or high levels of amylase?

   High amylase levels are expected, since a pseudocyst is essentially a contained leak of the pancreatic duct, resulting from pancreatic necrosis.

8. What is a **Sister Mary Joseph nodule**?

   A palpable firm nodule in the umbilicus indicating the presence of carcinomatosis, most often seen in patients with pancreatic or gastric cancer.

9. What is a **Trousseau sign**?

   Dr. Trousseau reported on the phenomenon of migratory venous thrombosis seen in patients with advanced malignancies, and realized that cancer represented a hypercoagulable state. He later noted the sign in himself and died of pancreatic cancer within a few months.

Pancreatectomy

Pancreatic adenocarcinoma

- The majority of patients present with metastatic or locally unresectable disease
- Lesions in head tend to present at earlier stages since the tumor obstructs the common bile duct causing jaundice
- Body/tail lesions present late, when local invasion into the celiac plexus causes back pain
- Tumor marker: CA 19-9
- Courvoisier's sign: palpable, distended, non-tender gallbladder, due to progressive distal obstruction

Cystic neoplasms

- Intraductal papillary mucinous neoplasm
- Mucinous cystic neoplasm
- Serous cystic neoplasm
- Pseudocysts

Pancreatic endocrine tumors

- Insulinoma: usually benign, evenly distributed through pancreas, presents with hypoglycemia
- Gastrinoma: usually malignant, located in duodenum or head of pancreas, presents with fulminant ulcer disease associated with MEN syndrome
- VIPoma: rare, usually malignant, presents with massive secretory diarrhea
- Glucagonoma: rare, malignant, presents with diabetes, dermatitis, and deep venous thrombosis
- Somatostatinoma: rarest, non-specific symptoms
- Non-functioning tumor: size, location, and aggres siveness varies, often found incidentally

Technique: Whipple procedure
- Diagnostic laparoscopy
- Lowering of hepatic flexure of colon
- Duodenal mobilization with Kocher maneuver
- Identification of superior mesenteric vein at inferior border of pancreas
- Cholecystectomy
- Hilar dissection with ligation of gastroduodenal artery and transection of common bile duct
- Establish tunnel between superior mesenteric vein and portal vein
- Transection of the distal stomach and jejunum
- Transection of the pancreatic neck
- Dissection of the uncinate process off the superior mesenteric vein and artery
- Reconstruction with 3 anastomoses: hepaticojejunostomy, pancreaticojejunostomy, gastrojejunostomy (alternative: pylorus-preserving duodenojejunostomy)

Technique: Distal pancreatectomy
- Diagnostic laparoscopy
- Entry into lesser sac
- Identification of point of transection based on location of lesion
- Ligation of splenic artery and splenic vein if splenectomy is required
- Transection of the pancreatic body
- Dissection of retroperitoneal attachments

Peri-op orders
- Pre-incision antibiotics
- NPO, advance diet as tolerated
- Drain output monitoring
- Trivalent vaccine if splenectomy was performed with distal pancreatectomy

Complications
- Hemorrhage
- Pancreatic leak occurs in up to 1/3rd of patients, but only the minority of leaks are clinically significant, rarely requires reoperation

Suggested Readings

Kennedy EP, Brody JR, Yeo CJ. Neoplasms of the endocrine pancreas. In: Mulholland MW, Lillemoe KD, Doherty GM, Maier RV, Simeone DM, Upchurch GR, editors. Greenfield's surgery scientific principles and practice. 5th ed. Philadelphia: Lippincott Williams & Wilkins; 2011.

Bose D, Katz MHG, Fleming JB. Pancreatic adenocarcinoma. In: Feig BW, editor. The MD Anderson surgical oncology handbook. 5th ed. Philadelphia: Lippincott Williams & Wilkins; 2012.

10
Splenectomy

Introduction

Splenectomy, or removal of the spleen, may be indicated for a variety of disorders, with traumatic injury to this organ being the most common indication for surgery. Despite its relatively protected position behind the ribs, the spleen is still susceptible to injury from blunt and penetrating trauma. In addition, rapid deceleration, such as occurs from falls, can avulse the spleen from its attachments and cause bleeding. Since the spleen is a highly vascular organ, splenic injury can lead to life-threatening exsanguination (Fig. 10.1).

While minor injuries can be treated non-operatively, deep fractures through the parenchyma require prompt intervention. Coil embolization of the splenic artery by interventional radiology is a less invasive alternative to splenectomy in the relatively stable trauma patient. However, persistent transfusion requirements or profound hemodynamic instability are indications for immediate surgery. In the OR, simple splenectomy is the most expeditious way to control hemorrhage. However, splenic salvage can be attempted with **splenorrhaphy**, wherein an absorbable mesh is used to tightly wrap the spleen, allowing for tamponade and hemostasis. This approach should be particularly considered for pediatric patients, in whom splenic function is physiologically more important than adults. When an injured spleen has been managed either by splenorrhaphy or embolization, it is important to remember

U. Sarpel, *Surgery: An Introductory Guide*,
DOI 10.1007/978-1-4939-0903-2_10,
© Springer Science+Business Media New York 2014

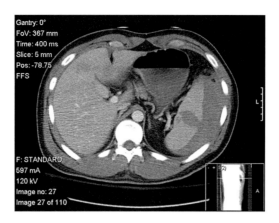

F<small>IG</small>. 10.1 CT scan findings in a trauma patient demonstrating a splenic laceration with surrounding hemoperitoneum

that delayed splenic rupture can occur up to 2 weeks after the initial insult.

Splenectomy is also often indicated for the treatment of certain hematological disorders. Historically, splenectomy was routinely performed to stage patients with Hodgkin's lymphoma, although the development of high-resolution CT scans has made this only rarely necessary. Currently, the most common indication for elective splenectomy is for the treatment of **idiopathic thrombocytopenic purpura** (ITP). This disorder, which is thought to be due to the production of antiplatelet antibodies, causes increased platelet destruction along with decreased platelet production, resulting in marked **thrombocytopenia**. Steroid therapy is the first line of treatment, however some patients will relapse after completion of their steroid course. Splenectomy is ultimately necessary in most patients refractory to medical therapy. When performing splenectomy for ITP, a diligent search for **accessory spleens** must also be conducted (Figs. 10.2 and 10.3). If such accessory spleens are inadvertently left in situ, they will hypertrophy and cause recurrence of the ITP. Following splenectomy, most patients with ITP will achieve a durable, complete remission with normalization of their platelet counts.

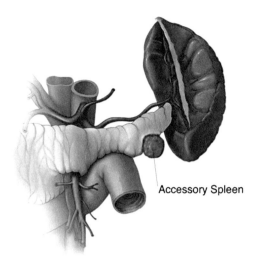

Accessory Spleen

Fig. 10.2 Accessory spleen closely associated with the tail of the pancreas. [Reprinted from Kawamoto S, Johnson PT, Hall H, et al. Intrapancreatic accessory spleen: CT appearance and differential diagnosis. Abdominal Imaging 2012; 37(5): 812-827. With permission from Springer Verlag]

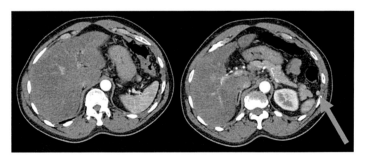

Fig. 10.3 CT scan image of a patient with an accessory spleen lateral to the spleen (*arrow*)

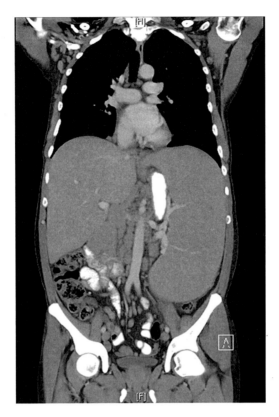

FIG. 10.4 Coronal CT scan image demonstrating massive splenomegaly

Splenectomy may also occasionally be recommended for thrombotic thrombocytopenic purpura, myelofibrosis, hairy cell leukemia, and other hematologic disorders, although this is less common. In some hematologic disorders, the spleen can be massively enlarged, making surgical resection technically more challenging (Fig. 10.4).

Another indication for splenectomy is for the treatment of **gastric varices** that occur as a result of **splenic vein thrombosis**. Spontaneous thrombosis of the splenic vein most commonly occurs due to an episode of pancreatitis. The intense inflammation associated with process causes irritation of the

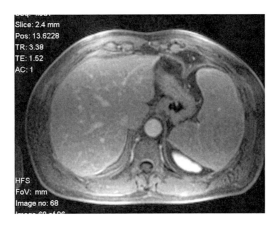

FIG. 10.5 CT scan demonstrating a mass lesion in the splenic parenchyma

splenic vein running along the body of the pancreas, and ultimately leads to thrombosis of this vessel. Arterial blood continues to enter the spleen but venous drainage is occluded, leading to **sinistral hypertension** and engorgement of the short gastric veins. Patients with such gastric varices can experience life-threatening upper gastrointestinal hemorrhage. Splenectomy is curative since it ligates the splenic artery inflow and divides the short gastric vessels to the stomach.

Occasionally, splenectomy is indicated when imaging demonstrates a lesion within the spleen (Fig. 10.5). The differential diagnosis of splenic lesions is long and includes primary malignancies and metastases, abscess, and infarct. These entities can be difficult to distinguish by radiologic criteria and splenectomy is sometimes the most expeditious method of obtaining a diagnosis.

Finally, splenectomy is often performed as part of a distal pancreatectomy procedure. This is most often the case when a pancreatic tumor in the distal pancreas encases the splenic vein, or encroaches upon the splenic hilum. In these situations, a splenectomy en bloc with the distal pancreas is indicated for both oncologic principles and technical feasibility.

Surgical Technique

Splenectomy can be performed by either an open or laparo-scopic approach. For open surgery, a left subcostal incision is typically used, although this should be considered on a case-by-case basis. For example, in patients with massively enlarged spleens, a midline incision may be preferred since the hilum of the spleen will be displaced towards the midline. A midline laparotomy is also best if splenectomy is being performed for trauma, since a subcostal incision is more time-consuming to perform. Once the abdomen is entered, the first step is to enter the **lesser sac** and then to divide the short gastric arter-ies. Next the **splenocolic ligament**, which connects the colon to the spleen, is divided. Once the stomach and colon have been reflected away, the pancreas and splenic hilum will be visible (Fig. 10.6). The lateral attachments of the spleen are divided, allowing the spleen to be rolled medially. Next, the tail of the pancreas is carefully dissected to reveal the splenic vessels.

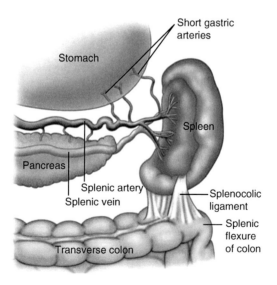

Fig. 10.6 Surgical anatomy during splenectomy: greater curvature of the stomach, short gastric arteries, splenic artery, splenic vein, sple-nocolic ligament, splenic flexure of the colon, and pancreatic tail

The **splenic artery** is ligated first, followed by the **splenic vein**. Alternatively, a vascular stapler can be fired across the hilum en masse, thus freeing the specimen.

Laparoscopic splenectomy begins in a similar manner to its open counterpart. The lateral attachments of the spleen are typically left intact until the end, since they assist in providing retraction and visualization. In cases of splenectomy for benign diseases, **morcellation** of the spleen can be performed, allowing even massive spleens to be removed piecemeal through small trocar sites.

Complications

The classic pitfall of splenectomy is inadvertent injury to the pancreas. The tail of the pancreas lies nestled in the hilum of the spleen. Particularly during a harried trauma case, injury to the tail of the pancreas can occur, leading to a **pancreatic leak** and the development of a collection in the splenic bed. For this reason, most surgeons will leave a closed suction drain in the left upper quadrant after splenectomy.

Another well-known complication of splenectomy is **inadvertent enterotomy** of the stomach or colon. The short gastric vessels that connect the stomach and spleen can be very short in length. During the division or cauterization of these vessels, the surgeon can inadvertently cause an injury to the greater curve of the stomach. Similarly, colonic injury can occur during mobilization of the splenic flexure of the colon.

Longer-term issues include the risk of **overwhelming postsplenectomy sepsis**. Also this complication is much discussed, it is fortunately rare in children and even more so in adults, with an incidence less than 1 %. The spleen plays a role in the defense against encapsulated bacteria, and therefore asplenic patients are at risk for infection from *Streptococcus pneumoniae, Haemophilus influenzae* type B, and *Neisseria meningitidis*. Vaccines against these agents should be administered to all patients undergoing splenectomy, ideally at least 2 weeks prior to scheduled splenectomy. In addition, young children undergoing splenectomy are typically started on prophylactic antibiotics.

Classic Case

A 16-year-old male is playing high-school football and is tackled from the left side. The patient arrives in the emergency department and complains of left shoulder pain. He is tachycardic to 112 bpm, but is normotensive. The abdomen is mildly tender on exam. Abdominal sonography reveals free fluid in the abdomen. A CT scan reveals a splenic fracture, with extravasation of intravenous contrast. Emergent coil embolization of the splenic artery is performed. The patient receives two units of packed red blood cells and his heart rate returns to normal. The patient is discharged home with instructions to avoid contact sports for a minimum of 1 month.

OR Questions

1. When should vaccination be performed in the case of unanticipated splenectomy, such as for trauma?
   The vaccines may be administered 2 weeks postoperatively.
2. Following splenectomy, a patient develops a left subphrenic fluid collection. Interventional radiology performs a percutaneous drainage and analysis of the fluid reveals an amylase level of 5,800. What is the diagnosis?
   Injury to the tail of the pancreas with resultant pancreatic leak.
3. What is the most common location for accessory spleens?
   The splenic hilum.
4. What happens if, during splenectomy for ITP, the retrieval bag ruptures and fragments of the spleen fall back into the abdomen?
   The splenic particles can implant into the omentum, regain a blood supply and hypertrophy, ultimately leading to recurrence of ITP.
5. In a trauma patient whose splenic injury is being managed non-operatively, how many units of blood are considered the limit before splenectomy should be performed?
   Six units of packed red blood cells.
6. Which blood test will be abnormal following a splenectomy?
   Leukocytosis will be noted on a complete blood cell count; this is a normal finding following splenectomy.

7. What is the most common cause of thrombocytopenia?
Cirrhosis of the liver increases the resistance for blood flowing from the portal vein through the liver, into the vena cava. This portal hypertension results in the back up of blood into the spleen, causing splenomegaly, which in turn leads to platelet sequestration.

Splenectomy

Indications
- Traumatic splenic fracture
- Idiopathic thrombocytopenic purpura: autoimmune disorder characterized by thrombocytopenia, initial therapy is oral steroids, splenectomy is indicated for failure of medical therapy
- Gastric varices: secondary to splenic vein thrombosis, usually a result of pancreatitis
- Thrombotic thrombocytopenic purpura
- Lymphoma staging
- Myelofibrosis
- Splenic abscess

Overwhelming post-splenectomy sepsis
- Spleen plays a role in the defense against encapsulated bacteria
- Patients should be vaccinated against streptococcus pneumoniae, haemophilus influenzae type B, meningococcus
- Antibiotic prophylaxis may be recommended for asplenic children

Splenic trauma
- Commonly injured in blunt abdominal trauma or rapid deceleration injuries
- Minor splenic lacerations can often be managed non-operatively
- Coil embolization of the splenic artery is an option in relatively stable patients
- Splenorrhaphy with mesh wrap may preserve an injured spleen
- Delayed splenic rupture can occur two weeks post-trauma

Accessory spleens
- Most are found in the splenic hilum, greater omentum, and small bowel mesentery
- Failure to identify and remove an accessory spleen may result recurrence of ITP

Technique
- Laparoscopic or open approach via midline or left subcostal incision
- Entry into lesser sac
- Division of short gastric vessels
- Mobilization of splenic flexure of colon
- Division of splenic attachments to lateral sidewall
- Ligation of splenic artery and vein
- Morcellation of spleen for laparoscopic cases

Peri-op orders
- Pre-operative vaccination, if elective case
- Consider placement of closed-suction drain
- Clear liquids, advance diet as tolerated
- Vaccinations may be given two weeks post-splenectomy if not done pre-op

Complications
- Pancreatic leak due to injury of the pancreatic tail
- Inadvertent enterotomy to the stomach or splenic flexure of colon
- Subphrenic abscess

Suggested Reading

Park AE, Godinez CD. Spleen. In: Brunicardi FC, Andersen DK, Billiar TR, Dunn DL, Hunter JG, Matthews JB, Pollock RE, editors. Schwartz's principles of surgery. 9th ed. New York: McGraw-Hill Professional Publishing; 2010.

11
Small Bowel Resection

Introduction

A wide variety of pathologies can affect the small bowel and require surgical resection. Interestingly, despite being the longest segment of the GI tract, primary malignant tumors of the small bowel occur less frequently than other sites. The most common tumor of the small intestines is **small bowel adenocarcinoma**; other possible neoplasms include **carcinoid tumor** (Fig. 11.1), **gastrointestinal stromal tumor** (GIST), and **lymphoma** (Fig. 11.2). Metastatic lesions can also involve the small bowel, most commonly from melanoma or carcinomatosis deposits from other GI tumors.

Intussusception describes the condition where a portion of the small bowel prolapses over itself, similar to the way the segments of a collapsible telescope slide over one another. Intussusception causes intense crampy abdominal pain as the small bowel peristalses against the point of obstruction. The lead point of this process typically has some abnormality that initiates the telescoping. In children, that lead point is usually a Peyer's patch—an area of benign lymphoid nodules within the bowel wall. In adults, the lead point is almost always a malignant tumor. As a result, while intussusception in children can be managed non-operatively, in adults it is necessary to resect the bowel with its inciting pathology.

Crohn's disease is a type of inflammatory bowel disease of unknown etiology. Symptoms include chronic abdominal

U. Sarpel, *Surgery: An Introductory Guide*,
DOI 10.1007/978-1-4939-0903-2_11,
© Springer Science+Business Media New York 2014

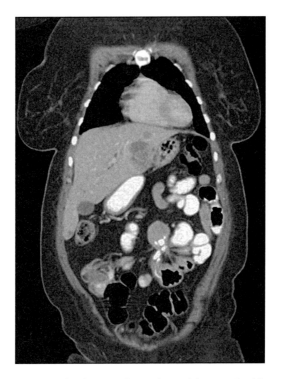

FIG. 11.1 Coronal CT image of a patient with a carcinoid tumor of the small bowel associated with calcified lymph nodes; also note the presence of liver metastases

pain, diarrhea, and weight loss. These symptoms can be accompanied by various extra-intestinal manifestations including ankylosing spondylitis, erythema nodosum, primary sclerosing cholangitis, and uveitis. Crohn's disease can involve any portion of the GI tract, causing aphthous ulcers in the mouth to perianal fistulae, but strictures of the terminal ileum are the most classic presentation. Multiple strictures may be present with skipped areas of normal appearing bowel in between. In the past, aggressive resection of all effected bowel led to many patients developing **short gut syndrome**. It is now recognized that resection does not prevent recurrence of Crohn's, and therefore **stricturoplasty** is the preferred

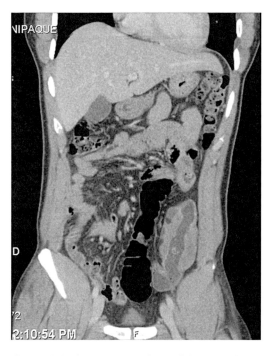

FIG. 11.2 Coronal CT image of a patient with a small bowel mass in the left lower quadrant; pathologic evaluation of the resection specimen demonstrated small bowel lymphoma

approach, allowing both relief of the stricture and preservation of bowel length. Bowel resection for Crohn's disease should be reserved for areas of severe obstruction, perforation, or fistula formation. Ultimately, Crohn's disease is a systemic illness and surgery can be used to manage complications, but does nothing to cure the underlying disease.

A **Meckel's diverticulum** is a congenital outpouching of the GI tract that occurs when the vitelline duct fails to regress completely. The "Rule of Two's" describes several classic features of a Meckel's diverticulum: it occurs in 2 % of the population, only 2 % of affected individuals will develop symptoms, presentation typically occurs before age 2, the diverticulum is usually located within 2 ft of the terminal ileum and is 2 in.

long, and finally—two types of ectopic tissues (gastric or pancreatic) can be found within a Meckel's diverticulum. The potential complications of a Meckel's diverticulum include intussusception, diverticulitis, or GI bleeding. These events are treated with resection of the portion of small bowel containing the diverticulum.

An **arteriovenous malformation** (AVM) is a focal vascular anomaly of the small intestine where there is an abnormal communication between local arteries and veins. These tiny lesions can cause spontaneous, intermittent, and massive GI bleeding. Often AVM bleeds are self-limited, however if there is continued hemorrhage, an emergent resection of the effected bowel may be indicated. Precise localization of the point of bleeding can be notoriously difficult. Intraoperative inspection of the small bowel is not useful, since the intestine becomes diffusely full of blood, and these lesions are not visible from the serosal aspect of the bowel. Capsule endoscopy, angiography, and intraoperative endoscopy can be utilized to help identify the point of bleeding.

Surgical Technique

Small bowel resection can be performed using either the open or laparoscopic approach, depending on the clinical circumstance and surgeon preference (Fig. 11.3). Once access to the abdomen is obtained, the area of pathology is identified and isolated. The normal intestine on either side of the lesion is transected, typically using a stapling device. If the enterectomy is being performed for an adenocarcinoma or carcinoid tumor, resection of the adjacent mesentery with its lymph nodes should be performed as well. Pathological analysis of the regional lymph nodes for the presence of metastatic disease will be used to stage the patient's disease and guide treatment decisions. When dividing the small bowel mesentery, it is important to avoid compromising the vascular arcade supplying the remaining portions of small bowel. The bowel can then be anastomosed in a hand-sewn

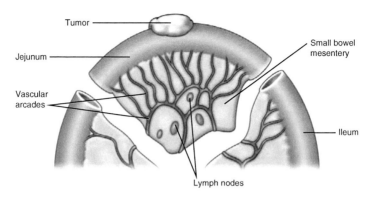

Fig. 11.3 Surgical anatomy during small bowel resection: jejunum, ileum, mesentery, vascular arcade, and lymph nodes

end-to-end, or stapled side-to-side fashion. The resultant defect in the small bowel mesentery should be closed to prevent an internal hernia.

Complications

One of the most serious complications of any bowel anastomosis is an **anastomotic leak**. Compared to the large intestine, the small bowel has a lower leak rate. As long as the segments of bowel being anastomosed are well vascularized and the anastomosis is free of tension, small bowel leaks are quite rare. If an anastomotic leak does occur, it may present with peritonitis, or — if the body has contained the leak — it may decompress through the skin as an **enterocutaneous fistula** (ECF).

An enterocutaneous fistula typically presents a few days after resection with what initially appears to be a wound infection. The wound discharge soon becomes enteric, establishing the diagnosis. The majority of ECF's will close on their own, although it may take several weeks of bowel rest and parenteral nutrition for complete resolution. The mnemonic "FRIEND" (foreign body, radiation enteritis, inflammatory bowel disease, epithelialization of the tract, neoplasm, distal obstruction) describes cases when an ECF is unlikely to close spontaneously.

While sometimes considered a complication, **adhesions** are part of the body's normal inflammatory response to surgery. Adhesions can occur after any intra-abdominal operation, although they are less common following laparoscopic surgery. It is unknown why some patients tend to form diffuse adhesions while others can have multiple operations and remain adhesion-free. Postoperative adhesions can lead to small bowel obstruction; the majority of these episodes will resolve in a couple of days with nasogastric tube decompression, bowel rest, and intravenous hydration. Patients in whom there is no return of bowel function after a few days, or who experience repeated attacks of adhesive bowel obstruction, should undergo surgical lysis of adhesions.

Short gut syndrome is the result of excessive resection of the small bowel leading to a malabsorptive state. The minimum length of bowel necessary to prevent short gut syndrome is approximately 2 m, but this varies significantly from individual to individual. Children are better able than adults to tolerate massive bowel resection since over time intestinal adaptation can occur allowing relatively normal function. A shorter length of small bowel can also be tolerated if the ileocecal valve remains present, since this structure helps to retain enteric contents in the small intestine longer, thereby facilitating absorption of nutrients at the terminal ileum. Tailored enteral diets have been created to maximize digestion, and total parenteral nutrition (TPN) can be used to supplement oral intake. Through GI rehabilitation programs, many short gut patients can be tapered off parenteral nutrition. Unfortunately, some patients remain TPN dependent, and a small bowel transplant may be ultimately indicated.

Classic Case

A 68-year-old woman presents to the emergency department complaining of abdominal bloating, nausea, and vomiting. She reports no flatus or bowel movements for the past 2 days. She denies any past surgical history or major medical problems. On examination, her vital signs are stable and she is in no acute distress. The patient's abdomen is moderately distended and tympanitic to percussion, but is non-tender to palpation. No inguinal or ventral hernias are found on exam. Rectal examination is unremarkable, but a fecal occult blood test is positive.

An upright abdominal radiograph demonstrates dilated loops of small bowel with air-fluid levels, consistent with a small bowel obstruction. A nasogastric tube is inserted with return of 750 mL of enteric contents. Given that this is a primary small bowel obstruction, the patient is taken to the operating room for exploration.

Pneumoperitoneum is established and laparoscopic survey of the abdomen reveals many distended loops of small bowel, limiting visibility. A laparotomy is performed and the small bowel is eviscerated. The terminal ileum is identified and the bowel is run proximally. A 3 cm concentric tumor is identified at the point of transition, and is associated with mesenteric lymphadenopathy. The segment of small bowel containing the tumor is resected, along with the mesentery. The ends of the small bowel are anastomosed in a hand-sewn manner. The pathology reveals adenocarcinoma with nodal metastases. The patient has an uneventful recovery and is referred to medical oncology for adjuvant chemotherapy.

OR Questions

1. During a laparoscopic cholecystectomy on a 42-year-old woman, the surgeon encounters a Meckel's diverticulum. What procedure should be performed?
   Only the cholecystectomy. An incidentally discovered Meckel's diverticulum in an adult should not be resected, since the vast majority of individuals will never become symptomatic.
2. What is the mechanism of GI bleeding from a Meckel's diverticulum?
   Ectopic gastric tissue within the diverticulum secretes acid, causing ulceration and bleeding of the small bowel mucosa.

The ulceration frequently occurs in the section of small bowel opposite the diverticulum. Therefore, a simple diverticulectomy will not remove the point of ulceration; a segmental bowel resection should be performed to ensure resolution of the bleeding.

3. A patient with Crohn's disease is taken to the operating room for the treatment of small bowel strictures. Upon running the bowel, the surgeon finds three strictures separated by a few inches of normal appearing intestine. Should all three strictures be included in a single small bowel resection?

   No, a stricturoplasty should be performed at all three sites, thereby preserving the full length of small intestine.

4. Evaluation of a patient who presents with abdominal pain leads to the finding of a small bowel tumor. In the OR the tumor is found to be associated with bulky lymphadenopathy. Upon manipulation of the bowel, the anesthesiologist reports that the patient suddenly becomes hypotensive. What is the likely diagnosis and what treatment should be initiated?

   Judging by the response to manipulation, this mass is likely a carcinoid tumor, and the patient is experiencing a carcinoid crisis in response to the massive release of serotonin and other vasoactive products. An octreotide drip should be initiated to inhibit the release of tumor hormones, followed by resection of the tumor.

5. Following a motorcycle accident, a 35-year-old woman undergoes a CT scan to rule out spinal fractures. The spine is uninjured, but the radiologist incidentally notes an area of small bowel intussusception on the CT scan. The patient denies any abdominal pain, and is having normal bowel function. What should be done?

   Observation only. Intermittent intussusception occurs as a part of normal intestinal peristalsis and is occasionally captured on imaging obtained for unrelated reasons.

6. A patient with atrial fibrillation develops acute mesenteric ischemia from an embolus to the superior mesenteric artery. She is diagnosed promptly and taken to the operating room. Upon exploration, most of the small bowel is ischemic. A thrombectomy is performed with some improvement in the appearance of the small bowel. How should this be managed?

Bowel resection should only be performed on frankly necrotic bowel. Mildly ischemic sections of small bowel may still recover viability, and should be reexamined at a planned second-look surgery. Radical resection of small bowel at the outset will result in short gut syndrome.

Small Bowell Resection

Malignant tumors
- Adenocarcinoma
- Carcinoid
- Lymphoma
- GIST
- Metastases (melanoma, carcinomatosis)

Intussusception
- Telescoping of bowel onto itself
- Presents with crampy abdominal pain and bowel obstruction
- In children, usually due to lymphatic hypertrophy and may be treated non-operatively if can be reduced with air/barium enema
- In adults, there is almost always a pathologic lead point which must be resected

Crohn's disease
- Inflammatory bowel disease
- Etiology unclear
- Can involve any portion of GI tract from mouth to anus
- Terminal ileum is the most common site of involvement
- Perianal fistulae common
- Skipped lesions
- Spontaneous ECF from inflamed bowel
- Treat with anti-inflammatory medications
- Use stricturoplasty rather than enterectomy when ever possible
- Excessive bowel resection in the past left many patients with short gut syndrome

Enterocutaneous fistula

- Develop due to unrecognized inadvertent enterotomy or anastomotic leak
- Most ECFs will close spontaneously over several weeks
- Unlikely to close spontaneously if:
    Foreign body
    Radiation enteritis
    Inflammatory bowel disease
    Epithelialization of tract
    Neoplasm
    Distal obstruction
- A high output ECF can lead to nutritional wasting
- Operative closure of ECF should be delayed for several weeks to allow the intra-abdominal inflammation to resolve

Meckel's diverticulum

- Found in 2% of the population
- Only symptomatic in 2%
- Most symptoms are before age 2
- 2 feet from terminal ileum
- 2 inches long
- 2 types of ectopic tissue: gastric or pancreatic
- Can cause GI bleed, intussusception, or diverticulitis

Arteriovenous malformation

- Focal vascular anomaly
- Can cause sudden, massive GI bleed
- Localization of lesion can be difficult
- Small capsule endoscopy can be useful in between bleeding events
- Angiography or intraoperative endoscopy can be used to guide localization during a bleeding event

Short gut syndrome

- Results when too little small bowel remains to support oral nutrition
- Occurs when approximately <150 cm small bowel remains
- Even less small bowel (100 cm) can be tolerated if the ileocecal valve is retained, since this slows transit time of intestinal contents
- Some intestinal adaptation occurs over time, especially in children
- Small bowel transplantation may ultimately be necessary for some patients

Technique
- Laparoscopy or laparotomy
- Identification of lesion
- Division of bowel
- Division of mesentery
- Creation of hand-sewn or stapled anastomosis
- Closure of mesenteric defect to prevent future internal hernia

Peri-op orders
- Pre-incision antibiotics
- NPO, or clears as tolerated
- Await bowel function

Complications
- Wound infection
- Anastomotic leak
- Enterocutaneous fistula
- Adhesions
- Short gut syndrome

Suggested Readings

Bowles TL, Amos KD, Hwang RF, Fleming JB. Small bowel malignancies and carcinoid tumors. In: Feig BW, editor. The MD Anderson surgical oncology handbook. 5th ed. Philadelphia: Lippincott Williams & Wilkins; 2012.

Soybel DI, Landman WB. Ileus and bowel obstruction. In: Mulholland MW, Lillemoe KD, Doherty GM, Maier RV, Simeone DM, Upchurch GR, editors. Greenfield's surgery scientific principles and practice. 5th ed. Philadelphia: Lippincott Williams & Wilkins; 2011.

12
Bariatric Surgery

Introduction

The worldwide rise in obesity levels has led to an explosion in the number of operations performed for weight loss. Even with dietary and lifestyle modifications, most individuals are only able to lose about 10 % of excess body weight, and relapse is extremely common. On the other hand, bariatric surgery usually results in rapid and dramatic weight loss that can be long lasting. The appeal of bariatric surgery is clear, however these procedures can be associated with significant morbidity, making patient selection and education critical to surgical success.

The **body mass index** (BMI), which incorporates both weight and height, is a more accurate measure of obesity than weight alone. Most medical organizations support the use of bariatric surgery in patients whose BMI is greater than 40 kg/m^2, or in those whose BMI is over 35 kg/m^2 if additional weight-related comorbidities such as hypertension, diabetes mellitus, hyperlipidemia, obstructive sleep apnea, or osteoarthritis are present.

Bariatric procedures are able to produce weight loss by at least two distinct mechanisms. **Restrictive procedures** decrease caloric intake by creating a physical reduction in stomach size. Purely restrictive procedures have a limited duration of effect because over time the gastric remnant will stretch to accommodate a larger volume of food.

Malabsorptive procedures exert their effect by interrupting normal absorption of ingested calories. Most currently used bariatric procedures utilize both mechanisms: a restrictive component to initiate rapid weight loss, combined with a malabsorptive component to ensure long-lasting effects. In addition to these stated mechanisms, it is now increasingly clear that bariatric surgery induces profound metabolic changes via recently discovered hormones such as **ghrelin** that are involved in the feelings of hunger and satiety.

A number of different bariatric procedures exist, each with a particular risk/benefit profile that should be considered on a patient-by-patient basis. **Gastric banding** involves fitting an inflatable plastic cuff around the gastric cardia, thereby limiting the amount of food that can be consumed at one time (Fig. 12.1). The degree of gastric constriction can be adjusted by the addition or removal of saline through a subcutaneous port. This procedure is almost purely restrictive in its effects, and therefore has a limited ability to produce long-term weight loss. However the procedure is associated with a low rate of surgical complications, and—since no alterations in anatomy are created—is reversible with removal of the device.

Another bariatric procedure is the **sleeve gastrectomy**, in which most of the gastric body is resected, leaving only a thin channel of stomach (Fig. 12.2). This procedure also relies on restriction of food intake for its efficacy. However, removal of a large portion of the stomach has been shown to result in lower levels of circulating ghrelin. Therefore, some of the weight loss seen after sleeve gastrectomy is likely due a decrease in the sensation of hunger.

There are several types of gastric bypass procedures; the **Roux-en-Y gastric bypass** is the most commonly performed version of this operation. Gastric bypass procedures combine both restrictive and malabsorptive properties by creating a small gastric pouch that is then anastomosed to the downstream small bowel, thereby reducing the opportunity for caloric absorption. While advantageous for weight loss, bypassing portions of the small intestine interferes with the normal absorption of various vitamins and minerals. Most patients

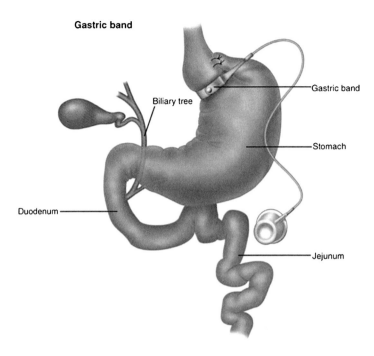

FIG. 12.1 Adjustable gastric band: a restrictive band is placed around the stomach thereby limiting food intake. The band is connected by tubing to a port that can be filled with saline to further adjust the degree of restriction. [Reprinted Perna MJ, Byrne TK, Pullattrana CC. Bariatric Surgery for Treatment of Obesity. In: Shiromani P, Horvath T, Redline S, Cauter EV (eds). Sleep Loss and Obesity: Intersecting Epidemics. New York, NY: Springer New York; 2012: 227-241. With permission from Springer New York]

who undergo gastric bypass require lifelong nutritional supplementation.

Patients qualifying for bariatric surgery typically undergo an intense preoperative program including a comprehensive nutritional assessment and psychological evaluation. Bariatric centers typically also require completion of an educational program that teaches about postoperative dietary restrictions and potential medical and nutritional complications.

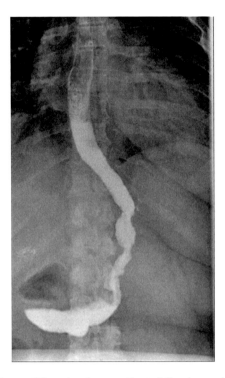

Fig. 12.2 Upper GI series in a patient following a laparoscopic sleeve gastrectomy; note the long, narrow channel of the residual stomach

Surgical Technique

Most bariatric procedures are now performed laparoscopically, which has the benefit of avoiding an incision in patients who are at high risk for wound infection due to the large amount of subcutaneous fat. Bariatric surgery is complicated by the difficulties inherent in operating on individuals with an obese body habitus. The process of establishing pneumoperitoneum is more challenging, and longer trocars and instruments are needed.

Once access to the abdomen is obtained, additional trocars are inserted. For laparoscopic gastric banding, the patient is positioned in steep reverse Trendelenburg to expose the left upper quadrant structures. The lesser sac is opened, the liver is retracted, and the upper stomach is dissected free of surrounding attachments. The band is inserted into the abdominal cavity, encircled around the gastric cardia, and secured into place with sutures. The tubing is brought out of the fascia and connected to the port. A subcutaneous pocket is created in the abdominal wall and the port is positioned into place.

For a Roux-en-Y gastric bypass procedure, the operation begins with the preparation of the Roux limb (Fig. 12.3). The jejunum is divided at the selected point and a downstream **jejunojejunostomy** is performed. The free jejunal limb is then brought up to the stomach in preparation for anastomosis. The stomach is mobilized and the gastric pouch is constructed using a stapler. The awaiting Roux limb is then anastomosed to gastric pouch, creating a **gastrojejunostomy**. The mesenteric defects are then closed in order to prevent a future internal hernia. Some surgeons perform an upper endoscopy at the completion of the gastric bypass to assess for any signs of an anastomotic leak.

Complications

The nature and severity of complications vary by the type of bariatric surgery performed. Laparoscopic gastric banding has the lowest rate of associated morbidities—most related to **slippage**, or **erosion** of the band. Perforation of the stomach can occur from inadvertent injury caused during dissection, but is rare.

The bypass procedures carry higher risks than banding, the most serious being an **anastomotic leak**. A leak can occur at either the gastrojejunostomy or the jejunojejunostomy, although the former is the more common site. It is important to note that physical exam manifestations of a leak such as tenderness and rebound are often blunted in obese patients;

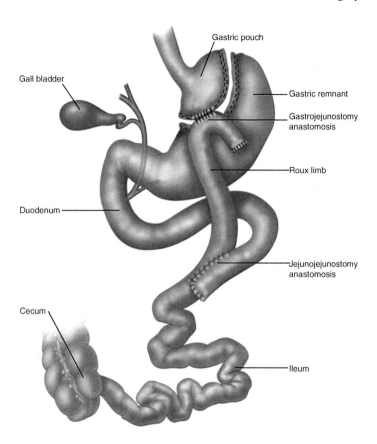

FIG. 12.3 Surgical anatomy during Roux-en-Y gastric bypass: esoph-
agus, gastric pouch, gastric remnant, Roux limb, duodenum, ileum,
cecum, gastrojejunostomy, jejunojejunostomy, gallbladder. [Redrawn
from Perna MJ, Byrne TK, Pullattrana CC. Bariatric Surgery for
Treatment of Obesity. In: Shiromani P, Horvath T, Redline S, Van
Cauter (eds). Sleep Loss and Obesity: Intersecting Epidemics. New
York, NY: Springer Verlag; 2012: 227-241. With permission from
Springer Verlag]

mild tachycardia may be the only objective sign of a leak. While anastomotic leaks are rare, they carry a significant mortality rate. Therefore, a high degree of suspicion must be maintained and postoperative tachycardia should be assumed to be a leak until proven otherwise.

Whenever a Roux limb is made, a mesenteric defect is necessarily created. If this defect is not closed, small intestine can become trapped within the opening, resulting in an **internal hernia**, known as a **Petersen's hernia**. Internal hernias likely occur more frequently following bariatric surgery because the associated weight loss results in greater laxity in the mesentery. Patients with an internal hernia typically present with symptoms of a small bowel obstruction. A high degree of suspicion and prompt surgical exploration is necessary before the trapped bowel becomes ischemic.

Patients with morbid obesity are at considerable risk for developing postoperative deep venous thrombosis and subsequent **pulmonary embolism**. Many bariatric surgeons routinely administer pre-incision heparin to reduce the risk of thrombosis. Ambulation on the first postoperative day is also an important measure. Any patient diagnosed with a pulmonary embolism should begin systemic anticoagulation.

Another potential complication of bariatric surgery is an **anastomotic stricture** at the gastrojejunostomy. Patients may present several weeks after surgery with progressive dysphagia and pain. An upper GI series showing anastomotic narrowing is diagnostic. Most strictures respond to endoscopic dilation, although multiple sessions may be necessary.

Long-term complications of bariatric surgery include **vitamin and mineral deficiencies** resulting from the malabsorptive nature of the operation. Most patients require lifelong supplementation to avoid nutritional deficits. Ultimately, **weight regain** can also be considered a complication of surgery. While bariatric surgery induces immediate weight loss, maintaining this relies upon patient adherence to dietary modifications, underscoring the need for a strong preoperative evaluation and educational system.

Classic Case

A 32-year-old woman with a BMI of 42 presents to a bariatric surgeon to inquire about weight loss surgery. She has tried several diets but has been unable to maintain any significant weight loss. After completing her preoperative evaluation, she is scheduled for a Roux-en-Y gastric bypass. The operation is uneventful. On the afternoon of the first postoperative day, the patient develops a mild, but persistent tachycardia around 108 bpm. EKG confirms that it is a sinus rhythm. The patient reports mild abdominal pain, but has no localizing complaints. Physical exam is unremarkable without signs of peritonitis. An upper GI study is performed with a water-soluble contrast agent and demonstrates free extravasation at the gastrojejunostomy. She is taken urgently back to the operating room.

At laparoscopy, a small defect is seen at the gastric anastomosis with some surrounding inflammation. The area is over-sewn and buttressed with omentum. Drains are placed around the site, and a gastrostomy tube is inserted into the remnant stomach for enteral feeding. Her postoperative recovery is smooth and she is able to reinitiate oral intake. The drains are removed and she is discharged home about a week later.

OR Questions

1. What effect does bariatric surgery have on a patient's diabetes?
   Most patients experience dramatic improvement in glucose levels, many with complete resolution of their diabetes. Interestingly, this effect is seen before significant weight loss has occurred, implying that the hormonal alterations seen with bariatric surgery likely play a role.

2. Why is a cholecystectomy often performed at the same time as gastric bypass?

   A significant number of obese patients already have gallstones; in addition, weight loss can further induce lithogenesis by changing the balance of bile composition. Therefore some surgeons advocate routine cholecystectomy at the time of bariatric surgery.

3. A patient who underwent gastric band placement 6 months ago reports new abdominal pain and fever. On exam there is blanching erythema and tenderness over the subcutaneous port site. What is the diagnosis and treatment?

   An infected port, most likely due to erosion of the band into the stomach, with tracking of enteric bacteria into the subcutaneous pocket; the gastric band and the port must be urgently removed.

4. Which vitamins and minerals require supplementation following gastric bypass surgery?

   The B vitamins (especially thiamine and B_{12}), vitamin D, folic acid, calcium, selenium, copper, iron, zinc, and magnesium can all become deficient after gastric bypass.

5. A patient who underwent a laparoscopic Roux-en-Y gastric bypass 2 years ago, with a resultant weight loss of 95 lbs presents to the hospital with abdominal pain, vomiting, and lack of flatus for 24 h. What is the diagnosis and how is it confirmed?

   While the most common cause of small bowel obstruction in a surgical patient is adhesions, an internal hernia must be ruled out in any patient who has undergone bariatric surgery. A CT scan of the abdomen can be obtained, however if the clinical suspicion is sufficiently high, operative exploration should be performed.

Bariatric Surgery

Indications
- BMI $\geq$ 40 kg/m^2
- BMI $\geq$ 35 kg/m^2 with obesity-related comorbidities: HTN, hyperlipidemia, diabetes, sleep apnea, osteoarthritis

Body mass index (BMI)
BMI = weight (kg) / height^2 (m^2)
- 19-25 = Normal weight
- 26-30 = Overweight
- > 30 = Obese
- > 40 = Morbidly obese

Mode of weight loss
- Restrictive: physical reduction of stomach size thereby decreasing caloric intake
- Malabsorptive: ingested calories are not fully absorbed
- Hormonal: decrease in the levels of appetite related hormones such as ghrelin

Types:
- Gastric band: solely restrictive, lowest risk procedure
- Sleeve gastrectomy: restrictive and hormonal
- Roux-en-Y gastric bypass: restrictive and malabsorptive

Technique: Gastric band
- Mobilization of upper stomach
- Band positioned and secured
- Placement of subcutaneous port
- Band tightness can be adjusted by addition / removal of saline via port

Technique: Roux-en-Y gastric bypass
- Roux limb is prepared
- Jejuno-jejunostomy is performed
- Mobilization of upper stomach
- Small gastric pouch is created
- Roux limb is brought up to pouch and gastro-jejunostomy is performed

Peri-op orders

- Pre-incision antibiotics
- Consider pre-op heparin
- NGT/NPO
- Upper GI study with water-soluble contrast
- Advance to staged bariatric diets

Complications

- Gastric band: slippage, erosion
- Anastomotic leak: gastric anastomosis most common site of leak, tachycardia may be only sign, potentially fatal, peritonitis may be difficult to detect on physical exam due to obesity
- Internal hernia
- Pulmonary embolism
- Anastomotic stricture: presents weeks after surgery, usually responds to endoscopic dilation
- Vitamin and mineral deficiencies
- Weight regain

Suggested Readings

Schirmer B, Hallowell P. Morbid obesity and its surgical treatment. In: Zinner MJ, Ashley SW, editors. Maingot's abdominal operations. 12th ed. New York: McGraw-Hill Professional Publishing; 2013.

Leslie DB, Kellogg TA, Ikramuddin S. Laparoscopic Roux-en-Y gastric bypass. In: Soper NJ, Swanström LL, Eubanks SW, Leonard ME, editors. Mastery of endoscopic and laparoscopic surgery: indications and techniques. 1st ed. Philadelphia: Lippincott Williams & Wilkins; 2009.

13
Enteral Access

Introduction

The ability to provide nutritional support to patients who are unable to maintain their own oral intake has dramatically improved surgical outcomes. Nutritional support should be considered for patients who have been NPO for several days, patients whose oral intake is insufficient to meet all of their caloric demands, and patients who are severely malnourished and require surgery.

Nutritional supplementation can be provided via the parenteral (intravenous) or enteral route. Unless specific contraindications exist, **enteral nutrition** is always preferable for several reasons: (1) enteral feeding is associated with lower rates of infectious complications; (2) enteral feeding does not induce liver dysfunction such as can be seen with parenteral nutrition; (3) enteral feeding prevents atrophy of the absorptive surface of the small bowel; (4) enteral feeding can be initiated immediately with nasogastric tube placement whereas parenteral nutrition requires central venous access and a patient-specific formulation; and (5) enteral nutrition is significantly less costly and labor intensive than parenteral nutrition.

There are several options for enteral access, beginning with the basic **nasogastric tube**. This is a good choice for patients requiring a short period of enteral nutrition. However, standard nasogastric tubes are made of a firm

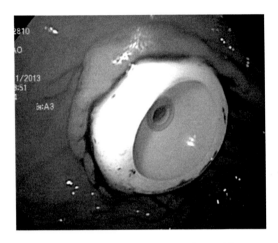

FIG. 13.1 Endoscopic image of a PEG tube in position

plastic that can cause pressure-induced necrosis of the nasal septum or alae. If nutritional support greater than a few days is anticipated, a smaller bore, softer tube should be substituted instead. Proper placement in the stomach should be confirmed prior to initiation of tube feeds with either aspiration of gastric contents or a chest X-ray.

Long-term enteral access options include endoscopic or surgical gastrostomy tubes. A **percutaneous endoscopic gastrostomy tube** (PEG) is the first choice, since it can be accomplished with sedation and local anesthesia, whereas a **surgical gastrostomy tube** (G-tube) requires general anesthesia. PEG placement is performed by passing a needle through the skin of the abdominal wall directly into the stomach, as visualized by endoscopy. Through a series of steps, this needle is exchanged for a guide wire, which is then attached to the PEG tube. The tube is pulled through the mouth, into the stomach, out the skin, and is anchored into place with a bumper on the gastric aspect (Fig. 13.1).

However, PEG tubes are not suitable for every patient. For example, endoscopic access to the stomach is not possible in patients with an obstructing pharyngeal or esophageal tumor. PEG placement may also not be possible in individuals with extensive prior abdominal surgery because adhesions may interfere with the ability to move the stomach into appropriate position. Proper PEG placement requires that the stomach be brought into direct contact with the anterior abdominal wall at a level below the costal margin. Failure to transilluminate the abdominal wall with the light from the endoscope suggests that other organs may be in the way. In patients who are not candidates for PEG placement, a surgical gastrostomy can be considered.

Aside from providing enteral access for nutrition, gastrostomy tubes can also be used for decompression of the stomach. For example, patients with carcinomatosis may develop intractable bowel obstruction as a result of extensive tumor deposits. A palliative gastrostomy tube allows for **gastric decompression** and is more comfortable than a long-term nasogastric tube.

A **jejunostomy tube** (J-tube) provides an alternate route for enteral access that may be more appropriate in certain situations. For example, some patients experience significant esophageal reflux and/or recurrent aspiration with gastric feeding. Jejunal access eliminates this problem by delivering the feeds distal to the pylorus. The downside of jejunostomy tubes is that they typically require surgical placement. Although endoscopic placement of a jejunostomy tube is possible, it is a technically demanding procedure only performed at select centers.

Once enteral access has been established, tube feeds are initiated and titrated up to the goal rate, as calculated by the patient's weight and caloric requirements. There are currently numerous versions of enteric feeds commercially available, including formulations for diabetics, patients with renal failure, and those with specific metabolic requirements. Close collaboration with a nutritionist is useful in order to select the appropriate formula and goal rate.

Surgical Technique

Open placement of a gastrostomy tube is performed via a small upper midline incision. Once the abdomen is entered, the stomach is grasped and an appropriate site on the anterior wall of the stomach is identified (Fig. 13.2). The G-tube should be situated in the midportion of the gastric body, away from the gastroepiploic arcade in order to prevent erosion into one of these vessels. Two concentric purse-string sutures are placed at the intended site and electrocautery is used to create a gastrostomy in the center. A large-bore tube with a mushroom tip or bumper is inserted into the gastric opening and the purse-string sutures are serially tied, thereby invaginating the gastric wall around the tube. The distal end of the tube is brought out of the body through a stab incision in the left upper quadrant. Four tacking sutures are placed around the gastrostomy tube to secure the stomach to the

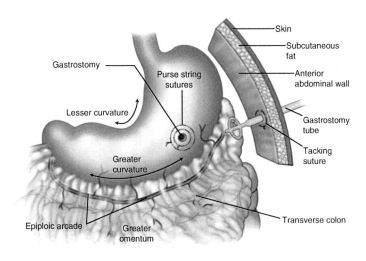

FIG. 13.2 Surgical anatomy for placement of a gastrostomy tube: greater curvature of stomach, epiploic artery, greater omentum, and transverse colon

anterior abdominal wall. The stomach is then brought flush against the abdominal wall and the sutures are tied. Saline is instilled into the stomach through the G-tube to confirm patency and rule out a leak. The abdominal fascia is closed and the gastrostomy tube is secured to the skin with drain stitches.

A jejunostomy tube is performed laparoscopically, or via a small midline incision. Once the abdomen is entered, the transverse colon is retracted, allowing identification of the Ligament of Treitz at the base of the mesocolon. The first segment of jejunum that easily reaches the anterior abdominal wall is brought into the surgical field. A single purse-string suture is placed on the antimesenteric aspect of the chosen loop of bowel, and electrocautery is used to create the enterotomy. A rubber catheter is inserted into the jejunum and passed several centimeters downstream. The purse-string is then tied, securing the J-tube in place. Most surgeons prefer to dunk the J-tube along the small bowel for a distance of 5–10 cm in order to decrease the chance of a leak. Interrupted seromuscular sutures are placed longitudinally along the tract of the tube and gently tied down, thereby burying the J-tube in a tunnel. The distal end of the jejunostomy tube is then brought out through a small incision in the left mid-abdomen. Several tacking sutures are used to secure the J-tube along the anterior abdominal wall. Saline is used to interrogate the J-tube's patency. The fascia is closed and the tube is secured to the skin with drain stitches.

Complications

Like any other surgical procedure that violates the integrity of the bowel, a leak is the most serious complication of enteral access procedures. Spillage of tube feeds or enteric contents into the abdominal cavity leads to peritonitis and sepsis. Close apposition of the gastrostomy or jejunostomy site to the anterior abdominal wall is critical to seal off the enterotomy and prevent a leak.

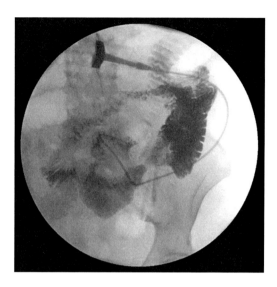

FIG. 13.3 Fluoroscopic image of contrast being injected into a jejunostomy tube to confirm proper placement

Another potential complication of a jejunostomy tube is
torsion of the small bowel around the point of fixation to the
anterior abdominal wall. This potentially devastating complication should be suspected in any patient with a jejunostomy
who presents with sudden abdominal pain and bowel obstruction. Urgent surgical exploration is necessary to reduce the
volvulus before the involved small bowel becomes ischemic.

Finally, **tube dislodgement** is a common complication of
enteral access procedures. Management of a tube that has
fallen out depends on the length of time since its placement.
The tract from the skin to the bowel becomes well established after approximately 2 weeks. After this time period,
the tube can simply be guided through the tract, and its position confirmed by X-ray and enteric contrast. However,
recently placed tubes may have only tenuous adhesions in
place, and blind reinsertion may avulse the bowel from the
abdominal wall. In this setting, interrogation of the tract by
interventional radiology is the safest method of establishing
tube position (Fig. 13.3).

Classic Case

An 82-year-old man with gastric cancer undergoes a total gastrectomy with esophagojejunostomy. His postoperative course is complicated by an anastomotic leak with resultant sepsis. He is taken back to the operating room where a small hole in the anastomosis is discovered. The site is suture repaired, drains are placed, and a feeding jejunostomy is created. The patient remains in critical condition, requiring a prolonged stay in the intensive care unit. During this period, jejunostomy feeds are initiated and titrated up to goal rate.

He slowly recovers and is able to be weaned off the ventilator. He initially fails a swallow evaluation due to aspiration, but is ultimately able to resume oral intake. The tube feeds are continued until he is able to meet all of his caloric needs by mouth. The patient is discharged to a rehabilitation facility where he undergoes physical therapy and is eventually able to return home. On outpatient follow-up, the jejunostomy tube is removed and the site is allowed to close.

OR Questions

1. Which organs are most commonly injured inadvertently during PEG placement?
   Transverse colon, left lateral lobe of the liver.
2. What are situations where parenteral nutrition is favored over enteral nutrition?
   Bowel obstruction, enterocutaneous fistula, prolonged ileus, abdominal sepsis.
3. Which is better, a G-tube or a J-tube?
   When clinically appropriate, a gastrostomy tube is generally preferable because it's placement is easier. A G-tube also allows for bolus feeds whereas jejunostomy feeds must be delivered slowly over a period of several hours since the jejunum cannot accommodate large volumes.
4. One day after open gastrostomy tube placement, while being rolled in bed, a patient's G-tube is accidentally

dislodged. The patient soon becomes tachycardic and complains of abdominal pain. What is the next step in management?

The gastrostomy site is likely leaking enteric contents into the abdomen. The patient should be taken emergently back to the OR for reinsertion of the G-tube and reinforcement of the gastrostomy site.

Enteral Access

Introduction
- Consider nutritional support for patients who are unable to meet their caloric needs by mouth
- Enteral nutrition is preferred over parenteral nutrition whenever clinically appropriate
- Enteral nutrition is associated with fewer complications such as infection or liver dysfunction, prevents atrophy of intestinal villi, and is less costly

Percutaneous endoscopic gastrostomy tube
- Less invasive than surgical G/J-tube
- Does not require general anesthesia
- Patients with obstructing esophageal lesions, or extensive past surgical history may not be candidates for PEG placement

Tube selection
- A nasogastric tube can be used for initiation of enteral feeds, but long term use is associated with alar necrosis
- Generally gastrostomy tubes are preferred over jejunostomy tubes since bolus feeds can be delivered, however gastric feeds may be associated with aspiration
- PEG and G-tubes should be avoided in cases where the stomach may be used as a future conduit following esophagectomy

Technique: Gastrostomy tube
- Appropriate site on greater curve of stomach is identified
- Concentric purse string sutures are placed at site
- Gastrostomy and tube insertion
- Stomach is tacked to abdominal wall

Technique: Jejunostomy tube
- Proximal jejunum is identified
- A purse string suture is placed on the antimesenteric aspect of bowel
- Enterotomy created and tube is inserted
- Tube is buried for 5-10 cm along jejunum
- Jejunum is broadly tacked to anterior abdominal wall to prevent torsion

Peri-op orders
- Pre-incision antibiotics
- Nutrition consultation
- Initiation of tube feeds
- Titrate up to caloric goal

Complications
- Enteric leak
- Torsion of small bowel around point of fixation to anterior abdominal wall
- Tube dislodgement

Suggested Reading

Steiger E, Matarese LE. Enteral nutrition support. In: Fischer JE, Jones DB, Pomposelli FB, Upchurch GR, Klimberg VS, Schwaitzberg SD, Bland KI, editors. Fischer's mastery of surgery. 6th ed. Philadelphia: Lippincott Williams & Wilkins; 2012.

14
Colectomy

Introduction

Colorectal adenocarcinoma is the third-most common of all
cancer types, and is one of the leading indications for colectomy (Fig. 14.1). Most colorectal cancers arise from adenomatous polyps that become dysplastic, in what is known as
the **adenoma–carcinoma sequence**. The progression from
polyp to invasive cancer is a slow process, involving a series
of genetic mutations, and takes approximately 10 years. As a
result, screening colonoscopy with polypectomy, starting at
age 50 years is highly effective at reducing the incidence of
colon cancer.

Colonic tumors are generally asymptomatic in the early
stages. Classically, it is taught that right-sided colon cancers
present with blood per rectum, whereas left-sided tumors
present with a decrease in stool caliber, however this is not
always seen in clinical practice. Some patients may report
shortness of breath or fatigue due to iron deficiency anemia
brought on by occult bleeding from the tumor.

Once an endoscopic biopsy confirms the diagnosis of
colon cancer, the next step is to stage the extent of disease.
CT imaging of the chest and abdomen are obtained to evaluate for distant disease such as pulmonary or hepatic metastases. For colon cancers without metastases, patients proceed
directly to surgical resection. Adjuvant chemotherapy is
offered if nodal involvement is found on pathologic evaluation

U. Sarpel, *Surgery: An Introductory Guide*,   145
DOI 10.1007/978-1-4939-0903-2_14,
© Springer Science+Business Media New York 2014

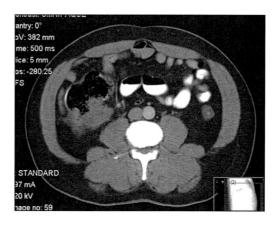

Fɪɢ. 14.1 Axial CT scan images of a patient showing a colon adenocarcinoma in the cecum

of the specimen, and in select node-negative patients with
high-risk tumors.

On the other hand, if metastatic disease is already present
at the time of diagnosis, most patients will be treated with
systemic chemotherapy only. In select patients with a small
burden of metastatic disease, resection of the primary tumor
and a **metastasectomy** may be considered. This approach has
been shown to prolong survival in well-selected patients with
colon cancer.

Occasionally patients with colon cancer present with **large
bowel obstruction**, due to a circumferential lesion that nar-
rows the lumen of the bowel. These tumors are called apple
core lesions, due to their imaging appearance on barium
enema (Fig. 14.2). Endoscopic stenting should be the first
treatment of choice for colonic decompression. If stenting is
not possible, a diverting colostomy can be performed to
relieve the obstruction. Resection of the tumor is not generally
recommended in this setting since the obstructed proximal
colon is dilated and may not be amenable to safe anastomosis.
Once the obstruction has been relieved, the patients can continue with the staging work up and treatment as indicated.

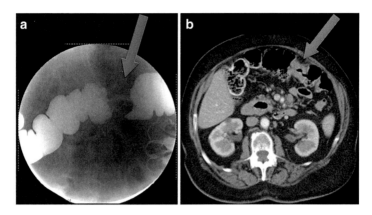

FIG. 14.2 (a) Barium enema and (b) corresponding axial CT images demonstrating a near-obstructing apple core lesion of the transverse colon (*arrow*)

Of note, colon cancer and **rectal cancer** have the same tumor histology and staging systems, however there are important differences in the treatment of these malignancies. Whereas patients with non-metastatic colon cancer proceed directly to surgical resection, patients with locally advanced rectal cancer should receive chemotherapy and radiation prior to surgery. This topic is described in greater detail in the section on rectal surgery.

The vast majority of colorectal cancers are sporadic, however there are also well-defined familial syndromes that increase an individual's risk for developing cancer. **Hereditary non-polyposis colorectal cancer** (HNPCC), also known as **Lynch Syndrome**, is a familial cancer syndrome caused by gene mutation and is transmitted via an autosomal dominant pattern. Patients with this syndrome are at high risk for colon cancer as well as several other cancer types including endometrial, ureteral, ovarian, and gastric cancers. Colonic tumors in patients with HNPCC typically arise without a preceding polyp, making endoscopic surveillance less effective. Patients with HNPCC characteristically have right-sided tumors and more frequently have synchronous or metachronous cancers.

Prophylactic colectomy is generally not indicated for individuals with Lynch Syndrome. However, once a colon carcinoma has developed it is recommended that the individual undergo subtotal colectomy at that time, to reduce the risk of future cancers.

Familial adenomatous polyposis (FAP) is caused by the loss of the APC tumor suppressor gene. The disorder is also transmitted via an autosomal dominant pattern; therefore, all family members of a diagnosed patient should also undergo screening. FAP results in innumerable colonic polyps that causes the near-certain development of colorectal cancer by the age of 45 years. Young individuals diagnosed with FAP should undergo prophylactic total proctocolectomy before age 25 years to prevent colon cancer development. It is important to note that in FAP the rectal mucosa is also at risk, and patients must undergo complete removal of the rectum in addition to the colon. Historically these patients underwent an **abdominoperineal resection** with **end ileostomy**. However, technical advances in surgery have led to the development of the **ileal pouch** that functions as a neo-rectum, and allows for preservation of bowel continuity. In patients with attenuated FAP who have rectal sparing, a subtotal colectomy with close rectal surveillance can be an option.

Ulcerative colitis is an inflammatory bowel disease that causes chronic irritation of the colonic mucosa, leading to abdominal pain and bloody diarrhea. Patients are initially treated with medications, however some individuals will have persistent symptoms despite aggressive pharmacologic therapy. Patients with medically refractory fulminant colitis or those who develop toxic megacolon should undergo urgent colectomy. Even with well-controlled symptoms, patients with long-standing ulcerative colitis are at higher risk for developing colorectal cancer. Close endoscopic monitoring is required to detect dysplastic lesions prior to the development of an invasive cancer. A biopsy of high-grade dysplasia should prompt surgery, since a focus of invasive cancer is highly likely. Similar to FAP, the rectal mucosa is at risk for

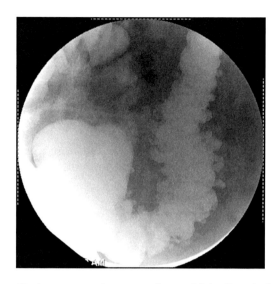

FIG. 14.3 Barium enema demonstrating multiple diverticula of the sigmoid colon

malignancy and must be included in the resection. Total proctocolectomy with ileal pouch—anal anastomosis is the standard operation for this disease.

Colectomy may also be indicated for the treatment of several benign processes. **Diverticulosis** is a condition wherein outpouchings develop along the wall of the colon, most commonly in the sigmoid region (Fig. 14.3). The incidence of diverticulosis increases with advancing age and may be the result of a low-fiber diet. Asymptomatic diverticulosis does not require any treatment, however two complications can arise from diverticulosis—bleeding or infection. Diverticula occur at the weakest points along the colon—the sites where blood vessels traverse the colonic wall. If one of these diverticula erodes into the adjacent blood vessel, acute lower GI bleeding will result. The hemorrhage associated with diverticulosis may be brisk and life threatening. Endoscopic control of the hemorrhage should be attempted first, but is often not technically possible due to the large amount of blood obscuring visualization. Angiography may be used to localize the precise site of bleeding, and the local delivery of vasopressors or selective embolization may be effective at halting bleeding in some patients. In the presence of exsanguinating hemorrhage from diverticulosis, an emergent colectomy should be performed. Segmental colectomy is acceptable if the source of bleeding has been accurately localized. In most cases, however, the site of bleeding is unknown and a subtotal colectomy should be performed.

Diverticulitis describes the infection that can occur if a diverticulum becomes impacted with fecal matter. Since most diverticula are located in the sigmoid colon, patients with diverticulitis will typically present with left lower quadrant abdominal pain and tenderness. This process may be relatively minor and resolve with bowel rest and antibiotics. Elective sigmoidectomy is generally recommended to patients who have had repeat attacks of diverticulitis. In severe cases, however, the diverticulum can perforate and result in **pneumoperitoneum** (Fig. 6.1). Patients with free air should be taken emergently to the operating room for exploration. If gross fecal contamination of the abdominal cavity is encountered, a **Hartmann's procedure** (sigmoidectomy with end colostomy) is the safest surgical option, since an anastomosis in the setting of infection is associated with a high anastomotic leak rate. Once the acute inflammation has resolved, reoperation to restore GI continuity can be performed.

Clostridium difficile colitis is an infection that occurs when antibiotic therapy disrupts the normal colonic flora, allowing overgrowth of one strain of bacterium. Patients typically present with profuse diarrhea, fever, and a history of recent antibiotic use. A stool sample should be sent to confirm the presence of *C. difficile*, however if the clinical suspicion is high, patients should be started on metronidazole or oral vancomycin empirically. In some cases, despite appropriate therapy, the disease can progress rapidly into fulminant colitis with multisystem organ failure. Patients who develop concerning signs such as hypotension or oliguria should undergo emergent subtotal colectomy without delay.

Surgical Technique

Various names exist to describe the different types of colectomy. A **segmental colectomy** is a nonspecific term that generally indicates a limited resection of bowel. An **ileocolic resection** is the removal of the terminal ileum to the ascending colon. A **right hemicolectomy** describes removal of the terminal ileum to the level of the transverse colon, and a **left hemicolectomy** refers to removal of the descending colon to the level of the rectum. A **sigmoidectomy** refers to a limited resection of the sigmoid colon and upper rectum. A **subtotal colectomy** is synonymous with a **total abdominal colectomy**, and indicates removal of the entire colon from the terminal ileum to the level of the rectum.

The above procedures involve the colon that is located within the abdominal cavity. The rectum exits the abdomen in the pelvis and is extraperitoneal for most of its distance to the anus. A **low anterior resection** refers to removal of the rectum past this peritoneal reflection. A **total proctocolectomy** describes removal of entire colon, including all rectal tissue. An **abdominoperineal resection** describes the removal of the rectum en bloc with the anal sphincter complex. These operations are described in detail in the section on rectal resections.

When a colectomy is performed for cancer, it is important to include the adjacent mesocolon that contains the regional lymph nodes draining that area of colon. A minimum of 12 lymph nodes is required for complete staging of colon cancer. In order to remove these regional nodes, the mesocolon must be divided as low as possible, taking the vascular pedicle near its origin. This maneuver is not required when colectomy is being performed for benign etiologies.

All of the described colectomies can be performed open or laparoscopically. A laparoscopic right hemicolectomy and an open sigmoidectomy are described in detail below as representative examples of the colectomy procedures.

For **laparoscopic right hemicolectomy**, pneumoperitoneum is established and trocars are positioned per surgeon preference (Fig. 14.4). The small bowel is reflected away,

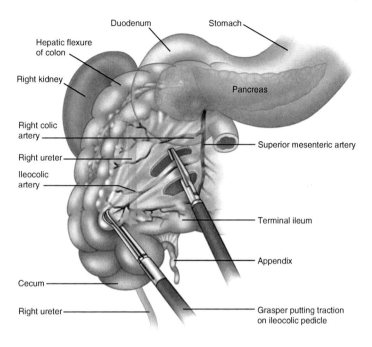

Fig. 14.4 Surgical anatomy during laparoscopic right hemicolectomy: duodenum, pancreas, terminal ileum, hepatic flexure of colon, cecum, appendix, superior mesenteric artery, right colic artery, ileocolic artery, and right ureter

allowing visualization of the mesocolon. The cecum is placed on traction, which causes the ileocolic vascular pedicle to become apparent. The peritoneum at this site is scored and the underlying vessels are isolated. These structures are then divided using a vascular stapler or energy device. A medial to lateral dissection under the mesocolon is performed until the abdominal sidewall is reached. During this maneuver it is important to protect the duodenum, which is located just beneath the plane of dissection. Next, the lateral attachments of the colon are divided from the cecum to the hepatic flexure; the lesser sac is entered and the dissection is carried to the transverse colon.

At this point, the colon is entirely mobile and ready for transection and anastomosis. Some surgeons perform these next steps within the abdomen, whereas others extract the colon from a small incision and perform these steps extracorporeally. The terminal ileum and the proximal colon are transected with a stapler, and the mesocolon between these points is divided with an energy device. The specimen is removed via a small incision and passed off the field. The two ends of the colon are aligned and anastomosed in a side-to-side fashion, most often using a stapling device.

For an open **sigmoidectomy**, the abdomen is entered through a midline laparotomy and the small bowel reflected upward. The lateral attachments of the sigmoid colon are divided, taking care to identify and protect the left ureter. The bowel is transected typically in the mid descending colon, or where clinically appropriate. The sigmoid is placed on traction which reveals its vascular pedicle containing the superior hemorrhoidal artery. This structure is ligated and divided. The inferior mesenteric vein is also identified and divided. A stapler is used to divide the upper rectum at the level of the peritoneal reflection, and the specimen is passed off the field. The proximal colon and splenic flexure are mobilized until the end of the colon reaches the rectal stump without tension. A circular stapler is then used for the anastomosis. The shaft of the stapler is inserted through the anus and its spike is delivered through the rectal stump. The anvil of the stapler is secured in the lumen of the proximal colon. The two ends are mated and the stapler is fired, creating the anastomosis.

Complications

As in all gastrointestinal operations, the most serious complication of colectomy is an **anastomotic leak**. Several factors affect the incidence of a leak. For example, left-sided anastomoses have a higher leak rate than right-sided anastomoses; a history of radiation is thought to increase the chance of an anastomotic leak; and an anastomosis created in an infected field is also high-risk. Technical factors that can increase leak rates are tension on the anastomosis and a poor blood supply to the tissue being anastomosed.

An anastomotic leak typically occurs after the fifth post-operative day, once the devitalized tissue becomes necrotic and breaks down, leading to spillage of enteric contents into the abdominal cavity. Some patients develop frank peritonitis, however more often the initial signs of an anastomotic leak are subtle. Sinus tachycardia, low-grade fever, persistent ileus, and a moderate increase in white blood cell count may be the early signs of an anastomotic leak. A CT scan demonstrating a fluid collection or air bubbles at the anastomotic site strongly suggest a leak. In general, patients with a significant anastomotic leak should undergo operative re-exploration and washout, and the proximal end of the colon should be brought up as an end colostomy. Other management strategies may be considered in clinically stable patients with a minor leak.

Another potential complication of colectomy is a **ureteral injury**. The left ureter travels just under the sigmoid colon en route to the bladder, and is at risk of injury if the plane of dissection is taken too deep. By contrast, the right ureter is more lateral in its course and is less frequently injured. Preoperative placement of ureteral stents can be a useful aid for cases where potential ureteral injury is of concern—such as in patients with severe diverticulitis or a bulky sigmoid tumor.

It is also possible to cause accidental injury to the small bowel or other segment of colon during the dissection and mobilization that is performed during the course of a colectomy. Electrocautery devices are the usual culprits of an **inadvertent enterotomy**, since the operator may touch a nearby loop of bowel without realizing that the device tip is still hot. Full-thickness cautery injuries lead to necrosis of the bowel, resulting in the spillage of enteric contents into the abdomen. Such burn injuries take a few days to break down into an enterotomy, and as a result patients will typically present with peritonitis several days after surgery.

Classic Case

A 72-year-old woman is brought in by ambulance to the hospital with a complaint of passing large amount of blood clots per rectum. Upon arrival she is tachycardic to 108 bpm and mildly hypotensive to 88/65 mmHg. She receives 1 L of normal saline, with little improvement in her hemodynamic status. Her hematocrit is found to be 23 % and a blood transfusion is ordered. She denies any pain and her abdomen is soft and non-tender. Digital rectal exam does not reveal any masses, but produces several maroon colored clots of blood. An emergent gastroenterology consult is requested. A colonoscopy is attempted, but is unable to visualize the source of bleeding due to the large amount of blood in the colon. An angiogram is performed and reveals active extravasation of contrast in the sigmoid colon. A highly selective embolization is performed with apparent control of the bleeding. However, 12 h later the patient begins passing clots per rectum again. Her repeat hematocrit is 24 % despite having received two units of blood and she remains tachycardic. She is taken to the operating room for an emergent sigmoidectomy. The bleeding resolves and she has an uneventful recovery from surgery.

OR Questions

1. What is the leading cause of large bowel obstruction?
   A primary colorectal cancer is the leading cause of large bowel obstruction, particularly if the patient is older than 50 years of age. *Other potential causes include colonic volvulus, and inguinal hernia containing colon, intussusception, or external compression from carcinomatosis.*
2. What is CEA?
   Carcinoembryonic antigen is a tumor marker that is often increased in patients with colorectal cancer. Although too insensitive to use as a screening test for the general population, CEA can be a useful way to monitor response to treatment and detect recurrence in patients whose tumors produce the marker.

3. What is the appropriate imaging surveillance for a patient who has undergone resection and adjuvant chemotherapy for a Stage III colon cancer?
   Most recommendations are for a CT scan of the chest, abdomen, and pelvis annually for 5 years. The risk of recurrence is greatest during the first 2 years after surgery and some physicians prefer to obtain imaging every 6 months during this high-risk period.

4. In a patient found to have colon cancer with numerous liver metastases, should the primary tumor be resected?
   Unless the tumor is actively causing symptoms such as bleeding or obstruction, there is no indication to resect the primary tumor. Surgery only delays systemic chemotherapy, which is the mainstay of treatment for metastatic colon cancer.

5. A patient with a history of intermittent left lower quadrant pain presents with a complaint of pneumaturia. What is the cause?
   Pneumaturia is the presence of air in the urinary stream, which indicates a colovesical fistula, most commonly the result of diverticulitis.

6. What is the "coffee bean sign"?
   Volvulus is a twisting of the colon around its mesentery, resulting in both large bowel obstruction and bowel ischemia. The dilated twisted loop of colon—most often the sigmoid—resembles a large coffee bean on abdominal X-ray.

7. What is in the differential diagnosis of a lower GI bleed?
   For massive bleeding, diverticulosis or a vascular ectasia (arteriovenous malformation) is the likeliest cause. More limited bleeding can be seen with a Meckel's diverticulum, colorectal cancer, hemorrhoids, ulcerative colitis, ischemic colitis, infectious colitis, and anal fissures. Also remember that the cause of blood per rectum may be from an upper GI source.

8. What imaging tests other than angiography can be used to localize the source of a GI bleed?
   A tagged red-blood cell scan is a nuclear medicine test that uses radiolabeled red blood cells to localize sites of active bleeding. Whereas relatively brisk arterial bleeding is

required in order to be visible on angiography, tagged RBC scans can detect slower rates of bleeding.

9. In patients being treated for *C. difficile colitis*, should vancomycin be given orally or intravenously?

   Intravenous vancomycin is ineffective in the treatment of C. difficile colitis because the drug is not excreted in sufficient amounts into the colon. Oral and rectal are the only routes of vancomycin administration that are effective against C. difficile.

Colectomy

Colorectal adenocarcinoma

- Adenoma-carcinoma sequence: progression from adenomatous polyp to invasive carcinoma
- Majority of tumors are sporadic, but some may be associated with a familial cancer syndrome
- Routine colonoscopy with polypectomy is highly effective at preventing colon cancer
- Symptoms: right-sided tumors often present with melena, or fatigue due to anemia; left-sided tumors may present with large bowel obstruction
- CT scan of chest and abdomen to rule out metastatic disease
- Colectomy should include the mesocolon to ensure at least 12 lymph nodes are obtained
- Adjuvant chemotherapy for patients with positive lymph nodes
- Survival may be improved by resection of limited liver or lung metastases in select patients
- Carcinoembryonic antigen (CEA): may be useful for monitoring treatment response and recurrence

Familial adenomatous polyposis

- Caused by mutation in the APC gene
- Autosomal dominant transmission with 100% penetrance
- Hundreds of colorectal polyps with near certain risk of cancer development by 45 years of age
- Extracolonic manifestations: duodenal adenomas, gastric polyps, osteomas, desmoid tumors
- The rectal mucosa is also at risk for malignancy and must be removed, therefore total proctocolectomy is necessary to prevent the development of cancer
- Attenuated FAP syndromes: patients have fewer polyps, may have rectal sparing

Hereditary nonpolyposis colon cancer syndrome

- Lynch syndrome
- Tumor may not arise from a preceding polyp, making prevention with colonoscopy less effective
- Older age of cancer onset than FAP
- Prophylactic colectomy generally not recommended
- Patients are also at higher risk for endometrial, ureteral, ovarian, and gastric malignancies

Clostridium difficile colitis

- Antibiotic use leads to disruption of normal colonic flora, allowing overgrowth of c. difficile
- Profuse diarrhea and fever
- Treatment is to discontinue causative antibiotic and initiate PO or IV metronidazole and/or PO or PR vancomycin
- Patients may develop fulminant colitis despite pharmacologic therapy
- Patients with signs of organ failure such as hypotension or oliguria should undergo emergent subtotal colectomy with end ileostomy

Ulcerative colitis

- Inflammatory bowel disease
- Process begins in the rectum and extends proximally into the colon
- Symptoms: abdominal pain, rectal bleeding, mucus per rectum
- Medical treatment: steroids and immunomodulatory drugs
- Indications for colectomy: intractable symptoms, then finding of high-grade dysplasia or carcinoma
- Colorectal cancer risk increases with duration and severity of disease
- The rectal mucosa is also at risk for malignancy and must be removed, therefore total proctocolectomy is necessary to prevent the development of cancer

Volvulus

- Colon twists on mesenteric axis, causing large bowel obstruction, and possible colonic ischemia
- "Coffee bean" sign on x-ray
- Sigmoid volvulus can be decompressed via colonoscopy, allowing elective surgery
- Cecal or transverse colon volvulus requires urgent surgical treatment

Diverticular disease

- Protrusion of mucosa through the layers of the colon, at the site of perforating blood vessels
- Sigmoid is the most common site
- May be related to a low-fiber diet
- Diverticulosis: no infection present, may present with massive lower GI bleed, emergent colectomy may be required if cannot be controlled by colonoscopy or angiography
- Diverticulitis: infection and/or perforation of diverticulum, presents with fever and left lower quadrant tenderness
- Simple cases of diverticulitis may be treated with antibiotics alone, contained perforations may be treated with percutaneous drainage, free perforations require emergent colectomy

Technique: Open colectomy

- Lower midline incision
- Mobilization of colon from lateral attachments (line of Toldt)
- Transect proximal and distal ends of bowel
- Ligate vascular pedicle
- Hand-sewn or stapled anastomosis

Technique: Laparoscopic colectomy

- Establish pneumoperitoneum
- Identify vascular pedicle to segment of colon and ligate
- Medial to lateral dissection
- Transect proximal and distal bowel
- Extracorporeal vs. intracorporeal anastomosis, per surgeon preference

Peri-op orders

- Consider bowel prep per surgeon preference
- Pre-incision antibiotics
- NPO or clears as appropriate
- Await bowel function

Complications

- Wound infection
- Anastomotic leak
- Ureteral injury
- Inadvertent enterotomy

Suggested Readings

Silberfein EJ, Chang GJ, You YN, Feig BW. Cancer of the colon, rectum, and anus. In: Feig BW, editor. The MD Anderson surgical oncology handbook. 5th ed. Philadelphia: Lippincott Williams & Wilkins; 2012.

Boutros M, Wexner SD. Concepts in surgery of the large intestine. In: Scott-Conner CEH, editor. Chassin's operative strategy in general surgery. 4th ed. New York: Springer Science + Business Media; 2014.

15

Appendectomy

Introduction

Acute appendicitis is one of the most frequent surgical conditions seen by the general surgeon and is the most common
indication for appendectomy. Appendicitis occurs when the
lumen of the appendix becomes occluded—typically by a
fecolith—leading to progressive distension of the distal portion of the organ (Fig. 15.1). Since the visceral peritoneum
lacks the ability to accurately localize pain, this appendiceal
distension first registers as a vague periumbilical pain. As the
inflammation progresses, the parietal peritoneum overlying
the appendix becomes irritated, which then localizes the process to an area in the right lower quadrant known as
McBurney's point. This migration of pain typically occurs over
the first 24 h of illness, and therefore classic right lower quadrant pain may not yet be present in very early appendicitis.

While patients of any age can get appendicitis, it is far
more common in children and young adults. It is important to
keep in mind that patients at the extremes of age have the
highest mortality from appendicitis, precisely because it is
unsuspected in these age groups, and the very young and very
old are often not able to describe their symptoms accurately,
contributing to the delay in diagnosis. If treatment is delayed,
perforation of the appendix can occur, leading to diffuse peritonitis and sepsis.

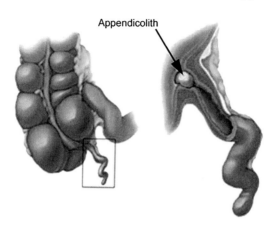

FIG. 15.1 Illustration of a fecolith causing obstruction of the appen-diceal lumen [Reprinted from Thompson SWS, Goldman SM, Shah KB, et al. Acute non-traumatic maternal illnesses in pregnancy: imaging approaches. Emergency Radiology 2005; 11(4): 199-212. With permission from Springer Verlag]

Typical physical exam findings associated with appendici-tis are **Rovsing's sign**, the **obdurator sign**, and the **psoas sign**. All three maneuvers elicit right lower quadrant abdominal pain by irritating the inflamed appendix, and their presence or absence can vary depending on the location of the appen-dix in relation to nearby structures (Fig. 15.2). It is important to note that several other processes can mimic appendicitis, particularly in female patients where pelvic inflammatory disease, tubo-ovarian abscess, ovarian torsion, and ectopic pregnancy must all be considered. Although in many cases appendicitis can reliably be diagnosed on the basis of a his-tory and physical exam alone, CT imaging has now become a routine part of the work-up. On imaging, the appendix will appear distended, thick-walled, and will not fill with oral con-trast; streaking in the periappendiceal fat indicates edema and inflammation (Fig. 15.3).

The treatment of appendicitis is almost always prompt appendectomy to remove the source of infection. However,

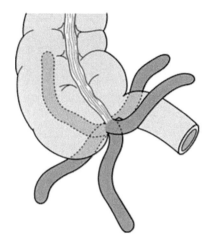

FIG. 15.2 Various locations of the appendix [Reprinted from Kosaka N, Sagoh T, Uematsu H, et al. Difficulties in the diagnosis of appendicitis: review of CT and US Images. Emergency Radiology 2007; 14(5): 289-295. With permission from Springer Verlag]

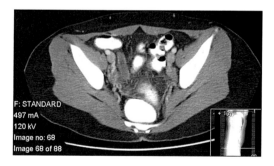

FIG. 15.3 CT scan demonstrating a distended, thick-walled appendix that does not fill with oral contrast, consistent with acute appendicitis

in certain cases of **perforated appendicitis**, it is more prudent to avoid the operating room altogether. In the setting of intense inflammation, the surrounding intestines become edematous and friable, greatly increasing the potential morbidity from an appendiceal stump leak or inadvertent enterotomy.

Therefore, it is occasionally appropriate to perform CT-guided percutaneous drainage of the intra-abdominal abscess and wait for the process to resolve while administering intravenous antibiotics.

Appendicitis in pregnancy deserves special mention. A pregnant woman with appendicitis may not present with classic right lower quadrant pain because the location of the appendix shifts upward with the increasingly gravid uterus. This feature—combined with the hesitancy to perform a CT on pregnant patients—can lead to a delay in diagnosis. If appendicitis cannot be confidently ruled out by the history and physical exam, ultrasonography and/or MRI should be used to investigate the diagnosis, since these modalities do not expose the patient to any radiation. "The morbidity of acute appendicitis in pregnancy is the morbidity of delay" is a surgical dictum that stresses the concept that it is not the appendicitis that threatens the patient and fetus, but rather the complications associated with a delay in intervention.

Although rare, the appendix can be the site of malignancy, including carcinoid tumors, mucinous neoplasms, and appendiceal adenocarcinoma. These tumors may present with appendicitis due to obstruction of the appendiceal lumen, or they may be discovered incidentally on abdominal imaging obtained for an unrelated complaint. **Carcinoid tumors** are a subtype of endocrine tumors, and can occur anywhere along the gastrointestinal tract, although the appendix is one of the most common sites. Small carcinoids at the tip of the appendix are sufficiently treated with simple appendectomy. Larger tumors require right hemicolectomy for sufficient margins and lymph node staging.

Carcinoid tumors produce serotonin, prostaglandins, and several other biologically active substances—however these compounds are largely inactivated by hepatic metabolism. **Carcinoid syndrome** refers to the episodic attacks of skin flushing, bronchospasm, and diarrhea caused by these substances when they are not inactivated by the liver and enter the systemic circulation. This syndrome is seen if the carcinoid tumor is located in an anatomical region not drained by the portal circulation—such as in the lung, thymus, or distal rectum. Carcinoid syndrome also occurs when the liver itself bears metastatic disease, allowing release of these vasoactive compounds directly into the systemic circulation.

Surgical Technique

Appendectomy can be performed by either an open or laparoscopic approach (Fig. 15.4). For open surgery, a small incision is made in the right lower quadrant over McBurney's point. Laparoscopic appendectomy requires a greater number of incisions for port sites, but has the advantage of visualization of the entire abdominal cavity. This is an important advantage if the appendix is in an unusual location or if the diagnosis is uncertain.

First, the abnormal appendix is located and dissected free of surrounding structures. Next, the **mesoappendix**

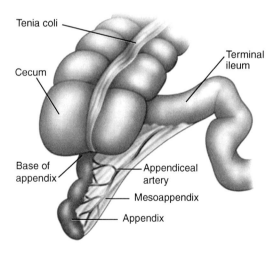

FIG. 15.4 Surgical anatomy during appendectomy: tenia coli, cecum, terminal ileum, base of the appendix, mesoappendix, and appendiceal artery

containing the appendiceal artery is ligated and divided. This exposes the base of the appendix at its junction with the cecum. It is imperative to divide the appendix proximal to the area of inflammation, through pink, healthy appearing tissue its base. If necessary, the surgeon should go lower to reach normal tissue, taking a small portion of the cecum with the specimen. Once the appendix has been removed, any purulent fluid in the abdomen should be suctioned out to prevent abscess formation.

Complications

The most common complications of appendectomy are infectious, including **wound infection** and **intra-abdominal abscess**. Rates of these infections are particularly high if the appendix is perforated. If an open appendectomy is performed for perforated appendicitis, some surgeons prefer to leave the skin wound open with a delayed closure in 4–5 days.

Patients who develop an intra-abdominal abscess classically present a few days after discharge with a fever. Diarrhea may also be present due to irritation of the bowel by the adjacent abscess. A CT scan will usually demonstrate a fluid collection in the pelvis with a rim-enhancing wall that often contains air bubbles, indicating the presence of gas-forming bacteria. Percutaneous drainage of the abscess cavity by interventional radiology in combination with antibiotics is usually sufficient treatment, and reoperation is only rarely necessary.

Classic Case

An 18-year-old woman presents to the emergency department complaining of abdominal pain for 2 days. The pain was generalized at first, but is now located in the right lower quadrant. She reports not eating dinner and currently does not feel hungry. Movement exacerbates the pain and she reports that during the car ride to the emergency room, the bumps in the road were particularly painful. She is sexually active and uses oral contraceptives; she denies any vaginal discharge.

Her vitals demonstrate that she is febrile to 38.6 °C and tachycardic to 104 bpm. On examination, she is lying very still on the stretcher. On palpation of the left side of the abdomen, she complains of pain in the right lower quadrant (**Rovsing's sign**). She tolerates slow, deeper palpation of the abdomen, but upon quick release of this pressure she complains of pain in the right lower quadrant (**rebound tenderness**). Pelvic exam does not demonstrate any cervical motion tenderness. Digital rectal exam is non-tender and negative for blood.

A CT scan reveals findings consistent with appendicitis. Antibiotics are administered and she is booked for surgery. A laparoscopic appendectomy is performed and reveals an injected appendix without evidence of perforation. She recovers from surgery uneventfully and is discharged home.

OR Questions

1. Where is McBurney's point, and what does it signify?
   The spot in the right lower quadrant that is one third of the distance from the anteriosuperior iliac spine to the umbilicus. It corresponds to the usual location of the appendix.
2. What is the arterial blood supply to the appendix?
   The appendiceal artery, a branch off the ileocolic artery.
3. A patient is taken to the OR with a clinical diagnosis of appendicitis. The surgeon finds a normal appendix, what should be done next?
   Appendectomy, and a search for other intra-abdominal pathology. The normal appendix should be removed to eliminate any postoperative and future diagnostic uncertainty.
4. A surgeon is performing a routine ventral hernia repair, should the patient's normal appendix be removed to prevent the potential for future appendicitis?
   No. A normal appendix should not be removed during an unrelated procedure. Even though the risks of appendectomy are low, complications such as mesh infection may occur.

5. During open appendectomy, a patient is found to have copious purulent fluid in the peritoneal cavity. Should the wound be closed?

   To decrease the possibility of a wound infection, the skin should be left open for a few days, followed by delayed closure.

6. From what types of cells do carcinoid tumors originate?

   These tumors arise from enterochromaffin cells, which line the digestive and respiratory tracts.

Appendectomy

Appendicitis

- Obstruction of the appendiceal lumen by a fecolith, lymphoid hyperplasia, or tumor
- Highest incidence in children and young adults
- Classic symptoms are right lower quadrant pain with fever, nausea and anorexia
- Patients lie still to relieve pain
- McBurney's point: 1/3rd the distance from the umbilicus to the anterior superior iliac spine to the umbilicus
- Pregnant patients may present with pain the right upper quadrant due to upward displacement of the appendix by the gravid uterus
- Patients with perforation are at higher risk for post-op abscess and wound infection

Carcinoid tumor

- Can occur in any portion of the GI tract, respiratory tract, or thymus
- May occlude the appendix leading to appendicitis, the diagnosis is often made incidentally on pathology
- Tumors secrete a variety of bioactive products, including serotonin and substance P
- Products are inactivated by hepatic metabolism
- Carcinoid syndrome: episodic attacks of skin flushing, bronchospasm, diarrhea
- Syndrome typically only occurs if the primary tumor is not drained by portal venous system, or there are liver metastases

Diagnostic maneuvers
- Rovsing's sign: right lower quadrant pain caused by palpation of the lower left quadrant
- Obdurator sign: right lower quadrant pain caused by internal rotation of the hip with a flexed knee
- Psoas sign: right lower quadrant pain elicited by flexion or extension of the hip with a straight leg

Technique
- Laparoscopic or open
- Locate and mobilize appendix
- Divide mesoappendix
- Divide appendix at the base of the cecum: failure to take the full length of the appendix may later result in "stump appendicitis"

Peri-op orders
- Pre-incision antibiotics
- Postoperative antibiotics only if perforation present
- Advance diet as tolerated
- Most patients can be discharged on POD#1

Complications
- Wound infection
- Intra-abdominal abscess
- Leak from appendiceal base

Suggested Reading

Doherty GM. Appendix. In: Doherty GM, editor. CURRENT diagnosis & treatment: surgery. 13th ed. New York: McGraw-Hill Professional Publishing; 2010.

16
Rectal Resections

Introduction

Operations to remove the rectum are most often performed for the treatment of rectal cancer. **Rectal adenocarcinoma** has the same histology and staging as colon cancer, however there are important differences in the treatment of this cancer due to the anatomical limitations imposed by the pelvic sidewalls and the anal sphincter complex.

Rectal cancer is loosely defined as an adenocarcinoma that is located within 15 cm of the dentate line. Once an endoscopic biopsy has confirmed rectal cancer, the first step is to perform a staging evaluation. A CT scan of the chest and abdomen is obtained to look for metastases, which most often occur in the lungs or the liver. **Pulmonary metastases** are more common in rectal cancer than in colon cancer due to the fact that the rectum drains directly into the systemic venous circulation as well as the portal venous circulation. Therefore, it is possible for tumor cells to spread hematogenously via the systemic circulation directly to the lungs, bypassing the liver.

Once metastatic disease has been ruled out, patients with rectal cancer require additional staging procedures to assess the local extent of the disease. Either an **endoscopic ultrasound** (EUS) or **pelvic MRI** can be used to evaluate tumor depth (**T stage**) and nodal involvement (**N stage**). Patients who are found to have early stage tumors proceed directly to

U. Sarpel, *Surgery: An Introductory Guide*,
DOI 10.1007/978-1-4939-0903-2_16,
© Springer Science+Business Media New York 2014

resection, similar to colon cancer. However, patients with locally advanced tumors ($T \geq 3$ or $N \geq 1$) should receive chemotherapy and radiation prior to surgery. This **neoadjuvant chemoradiation**, which is not used in colon cancer, has been shown to decrease the risk of local recurrence and increase the anal sphincter preservation rate. Surgery to resect the rectum is then performed 4–6 weeks following the completion of neoadjuvant therapy.

Following resection, patients whose pathology demonstrates node-positive disease will go on to receive adjuvant systemic chemotherapy, in order to decrease the chance of recurrence.

Those patients found to have metastatic disease already present at presentation usually begin treatment with systemic chemotherapy, but may be candidates for **metastasectomy** depending on their clinical situation. Resection of limited pulmonary or hepatic metastases has been shown to prolong survival in well-selected patients.

Two features dictate the type of operation used for resection of a rectal cancer: the size/depth of the tumor and its distance from the anal sphincters. In very early stage rectal cancers, it is possible to perform a **transanal excision** of the lesion. This procedure is reserved for early cancers since a local excision does not include any of the lymph nodes draining the region. Therefore, the only candidates for transanal excision are those patients in whom lymphatic metastases are thought to be extremely unlikely. General criteria for local excision are patients with small, superficial T1 lesions, who have no radiographic evidence of metastatic disease to regional nodes. Finally, the tumor must be located in the lower segment of the rectum to be accessible via transanal access. These criteria may be extended somewhat in patients with multiple co-morbidities who would be at high risk for major intra-abdominal surgery. Serial postoperative imaging and endoscopic surveillance is necessary in patients undergoing transanal excision in order to detect any signs of recurrence.

The majority of patients with rectal cancer will not be candidates for local excision and instead require formal

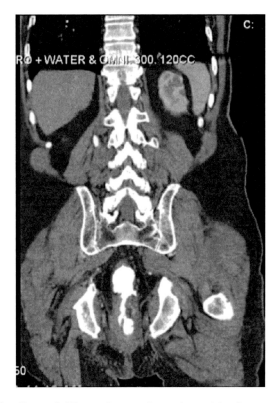

FIG. 16.1 Coronal CT scan image of a patient with a low rectal cancer involving the anal sphincters, requiring an APR

resection of the rectum. In most cases it is possible to resect the rectum and connect the proximal colon to the rectal stump, an operation known as a **low anterior resection**. This procedure maintains the continuity of the GI tract. However, for tumors located in the very lowest portion of the rectum, resection of the rectum en bloc with the surrounding anal sphincters is necessary in order to achieve tumor clearance (Fig. 16.1). This operation—known as an **abdominoperineal resection** (APR)—leaves the patient with a permanent colostomy, and is only employed in cases where sphincter preservation is not possible. This determination is heavily dependent on an individual patient's size, body habitus, gender, and pelvic anatomy. If the distance from the tumor to the top of the anal sphincter is less than 5 cm, it is usually necessary to perform an APR.

Whereas rectal cancer arises from the glandular mucosa of the rectum, **anal cancer** is a squamous cell carcinoma arising from the transitional or squamous mucosa of the anal canal. Rather than a sharp transition, these cell types overlap significantly over the length of the anal canal. Therefore, it is the histologic type that determines the classification and treatment of a tumor in the anal canal.

The vast majority of anal cancers are associated with **Human Papillomavirus** (HPV) infection. While some affected individuals develop anal condylomata, others may be asymptomatic and unaware of an existing HPV infection. Women with a history of HPV-related cervical cancer are also at higher risk for developing anal cancer. Of note, a history of hemorrhoids, fistulae, or fissures is not associated with an increased risk of anal cancer.

In the past, patients with anal cancer were routinely treated by surgical resection with an APR. However, it became apparent that non-operative treatment with chemotherapy and radiation provided the same survival rates without the morbidity of radical surgery. This regimen, known as the **Nigro protocol**, replaced surgery as the standard of care for the treatment of anal cancer. Most patients will demonstrate tumor regression with chemoradiation. However, salvage APR may be necessary in those patients who have residual disease after completing chemoradiation. Unfortunately these patients generally have a poor prognosis despite APR.

Surgical Technique

The rectum exits the abdomen in the pelvis and is extraperitoneal for most of its distance to the anus. A **low anterior resection** refers to removal of the rectum past this peritoneal

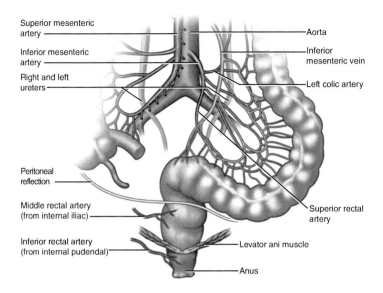

Superior mesenteric artery

Aorta

Inferior mesenteric artery

Inferior mesenteric vein

Right and left ureters

Left colic artery

Peritoneal reflection

Middle rectal artery (from internal iliac)

Superior rectal artery

Inferior rectal artery (from internal pudendal)

Levator ani muscle

Anus

FIG. 16.2 Surgical anatomy during low anterior resection: inferior mesenteric vein, aorta, inferior mesenteric artery, left colic artery, superior rectal artery, middle rectal artery, inferior rectal artery, levator ani muscle, peritoneal reflection, and right/left ureter

reflection. The terminology refers to the—now rarely used—alternative posterior approach to the rectum via removal of the sacrum.

A low anterior resection can be performed laparoscopically or open, with minor modifications in technique (Fig. 16.2). The abdomen is entered and the small bowel is reflected upward, out of the pelvis. The lateral attachments of the sigmoid colon are divided and the rectosigmoid is mobilized, taking care to identify and protect the left ureter. Depending on the amount of descending colon to be resected, the entire **inferior mesenteric artery** may be divided; alternatively, the **left colic artery** may be spared, ligating only the **superior rectal artery** branch. The proximal colon is transected at the indicated level and the dissection is carried distally. The peritoneal reflection around the rectum is scored and the lateral stalks containing branches of the **middle rectal artery** are divided. For rectal cancer cases, a **total mesorectal excision** must be performed, taking care to keep the mesorectal fascia intact. A stapler is typically used to divide the distal rectum. Next, in preparation for anastomosis, the splenic flexure is mobilized so that the proximal colon reaches the rectal stump without tension. The anvil of the stapler is placed within in the lumen of the proximal colon. The shaft of a circular stapler is then inserted through the anus and its spike is delivered through the rectal stump. The two ends are mated and the stapler is fired, thereby creating the anastomosis.

In order to test the anastomosis for any holes, the pelvis is filled with saline, and air is insufflated through the anus. If any air bubbles are seen when the anastomosis is distended, this indicates the presence of a leak. Depending on the clinical situation, the anastomosis may be revised, or simply reinforced with sutures. A **diverting loop ileostomy** should be strongly considered in patients with a positive **leak test**, or other risk factors for an anastomotic leak. A loop ileostomy is performed by creating a circular skin incision in the right lower quadrant of the abdomen. A cruciate incision is made in the anterior fascia, the fibers of the rectus muscle are spread apart, and the peritoneum is entered. The opening should be large enough to accommodate two fingers. A loop of the terminal ileum is then delivered through this opening and the bowel is opened. The proximal end of the bowel is matured into a **Brooke ileostomy**, and the distal end is sutured flat to the abdominal wall.

An **abdominoperineal resection** (APR) describes the removal of the rectum en bloc with the anal sphincter complex, and the creation of a permanent colostomy. This operation is performed via two incisions—one for the abdominal approach and the other for the perineal dissection. An abdominoperineal resection is begun the same as a low anterior resection and the dissection is continued distally to the level of the **levator ani muscle**. Once the dissection has been carried down as low as possible from the abdominal aspect, the perineal approach is started. An elliptical incision is made around the anus and carried through the soft tissues of the perineum until the levator muscle is reached from below. When the two planes of dissection meet, the specimen is freed, and is passed off the field. The soft tissue and skin of the perineum are sewn together to close the defect. The proximal portion of bowel is brought up to the abdominal wall and a permanent colostomy is created in the left lower quadrant.

Complications

A low rectal anastomosis carries the highest **anastomotic leak** rate of all GI anastomoses. By definition, the lower down an anastomosis is performed, the further the proximal colon is from its blood supply and the greater the amount of tension on the staple line. The use of radiation in the treatment of locally advanced rectal cancers is also thought to increase the chance of an anastomotic leak. If, at the time of the initial resection, the anastomosis is thought to be tenuous or there are other factors predisposing to a leak, a loop ileostomy should be created to divert the fecal stream until full healing of the anastomosis has occurred. The loop ileostomy can be reversed in about 2 months, once the rectal anastomosis is fully healed. The management of a patient with an anasto-motic leak is detailed in the section on colectomy.

Perineal wound dehiscence occurs commonly after APR. The adipose tissue of the perineum is poorly vascularized and therefore vulnerable to infection. In addition, pressure from the patient sitting on the surgical site contributes to the high incidence of perineal wound breakdown. Some surgeons pre-fer to use a muscle flap from the rectus abdominus or gracilis muscle to fill the perineal defect to aid in healing of this site.

Sexual dysfunction is an additional possible complication for men undergoing rectal surgery. Both sympathetic and parasympathetic nerve fibers course near the operative field and are vulnerable to injury. **Retrograde ejaculation** is the most common type of sexual dysfunction following pelvic surgery, and results from damage to the sympathetic hypogastric nerve fibers. This complication renders the individual infertile, however the condition may resolve with time. Damage to the parasympathetic nerves may result in **erectile dysfunction** and impotence, but this occurs less frequently. The incidence of postoperative sexual dysfunction can be decreased with careful dissection in the correct planes.

Classic Case

A 56-year-old woman presents to her primary care doctor with a complaint of bloody bowel movements for the past 2 weeks. She denies any weight loss or other symptoms. Colonoscopy reveals an ulcerated mass in the distal rectum. On digital rectal exam, the lesion is palpable at 7 cm from the top of the anal sphincters. A CT scan does not reveal any evidence of distant metastatic disease. An endoscopic ultrasound is performed and demonstrates a T4N1 tumor. She is referred to a medical oncologist and radiation oncologist for neoadjuvant chemoradiation. Repeat CT scans after the completion of therapy demonstrate tumor shrinkage and confirm no new metastatic disease. A digital rectal examination shows that the tumor is slightly smaller and of sufficient distance from the anal sphincters to avoid an APR. She is scheduled for surgery approximately 6 weeks after her last dose of radiation. An LAR with total mesorectal excision and a diverting loop ileostomy is performed. After recovering from surgery, she completes her adjuvant chemotherapy. The ileostomy is then reversed and she begins routine imaging surveillance for recurrence.

OR Questions

1. Does neoadjuvant chemoradiation for locally advanced rectal cancer improve overall survival?
   The data on neoadjuvant chemoradiation demonstrate a decrease in local recu3rrence rates and increased sphincter preservation, but no difference in overall survival.

2. Why does the remnant distal rectum not become ischemic when the inferior mesenteric artery is ligated during an LAR?

The distal rectum receives its blood supply from the middle and inferior rectal arteries, which are branches off the internal iliac artery, not from the mesenteric circulation.

3. Does a diverting ileostomy prevent a leak from an LAR anastomosis?

Probably not. However, by diverting the fecal stream away from the leak site, an ileostomy eliminates fecal contamination from a leak. This decreases the morbidity of a leak, and allows for non-operative management.

4. Are all strains of HPV associated with the development of anal cancer?

No, similar to cervical cancer, only certain strains of HPV have been shown to be oncogenic.

5. In high-risk patients with known HPV infection, is there any type of screening that can be performed to decrease the development of anal cancer?

Yes, anal pap smears can demonstrate areas of anal dysplasia. Areas of high-grade dysplasia can be treated with topical agents or with ablation.

6. In a patient diagnosed with anal cancer, which lymph nodes represent the first site of metastasis?

Anal cancer typically spreads first to the superficial inguinal lymph nodes. This is different from rectal cancer where lymphatic metastases tend to occur first to the mesorectal nodes.

Rectal Resections

Rectal adenocarcinoma

- Same histology as colon cancer, but with important differences in evaluation and treatment
- Endorectal ultrasound or pelvic MRI is used to determine T and N stage
- Small, distal, T1N0 lesions may be considered for local transanal excision
- Patients with locally advanced disease (T$\geq$3 or N$\geq$1) should receive neoadjuvant chemoradiation to decrease risk of local recurrence
- Distance of the tumor from the upper edge of the anal sphincters determines the type of resection (LAR if the sphincters can be spared vs. APR if the tumor involves the sphincters)
- Depending on body habitus, it may not be possible to preserve the sphincters if tumordistance is < 5 cm

Anal carcinoma

- Carcinoma of the transitional or squamous mucosa of the anal canal
- Associated with Human Papillomavirus infection
- HIV is a risk factor
- First line of treatment is chemotherapy and radiation (Nigro protocol)
- APR only used as a salvage procedure for patients unresponsive to chemoradiation, but is associated with poor prognosis

Technique: Abdominoperineal resection (APR)

- Mobilization of lateral attachments, transection of proximal colon
- Ligation of IMA or superior rectal artery as appropriate; ligation of IMV
- Total mesorectal excision to level of levator muscles
- Perineal incision and proximal dissection until abdomen is entered
- Extraction of specimen
- Primary closure of perineum, or closure with muscle flap from rectus abdominus or gracilis
- Closure of abdominal incision / trocar sites
- Creation of colostomy
- Colostomy is permanent and the site should be chosen carefully with regard to skin folds and body habitus

Peri-op orders

- Consider bowel prep per surgeon preference
- Pre-incision antibiotics
- Clear liquid diet as appropriate
- Await bowel function
- Stoma care teaching, if applicable

Technique: Low anterior resection (LAR)

- Mobilization of lateral attachments, transection of proximal colon
- Ligation of IMA or superior rectal artery as appropriate; ligation of IMV
- Total mesorectal excision
- Transection of rectum below tumor
- Mobilization of splenic flexure to bring proximal colon into pelvis
- Insert anvil into proximal colon
- Introduce stapler through anus and mate stapler with anvil
- Leak test
- Consider diverting ileostomy

Complications

- Wound infection
- Ureteral injury
- Sexual dysfunction: retrograde ejaculation, erectile dysfunction
- For LAR, anastomotic leak
- For APR, perineal wound dehiscence, colostomy necrosis or retraction

Suggested Reading

Bleday R, Brindzei N. Surgical treatment of rectal cancer. In: Beck DE, Roberts PL, Saclarides TJ, Senagore AJ, Stamos MJ, editors. The ASCRS textbook of colon and rectal surgery. 2nd ed. New York: Springer; 2011.

17
Anorectal Procedures

Introduction

Anorectal complaints are a frequent reason for a surgical consultation. The four most common benign anorectal disorders are: perianal abscess, fistula-in-ano, anal fissures, and hemorrhoids. A **perianal abscess** is an infection that occurs when an anal crypt gland becomes obstructed and cannot drain freely into the anal canal. The gland's infected products build up, resulting in a collection of pus in the soft tissues around the anus or rectum (Fig. 17.1). Patients typically present with pain and tenderness at the site and are often febrile.

In most cases an erythematous, indurated, fluctuant site is readily apparent in the perianal area. In certain cases, however, the abscess cavity is located higher within the anal canal and no findings will be seen on external inspection. For example, an **intersphincteric abscess** forms in the plane between the internal and external sphincters, and may only be appreciated on digital rectal exam as a tender bulge into the anal canal. A **supralevator abscess** is located even more proximally above the levator ani muscle. In this situation, a CT scan may be the necessary to diagnose the presence of an abscess (Fig. 17.2).

Treatment of a simple perianal abscess involves incision over the indurated area and drainage of the purulent material. A drain is left within the cavity to prevent the skin from closing over prematurely, which would result in recurrence of

U. Sarpel, *Surgery: An Introductory Guide*,
DOI 10.1007/978-1-4939-0903-2_17,
© Springer Science+Business Media New York 2014

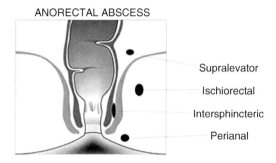

FIG. 17.1 Diagram of the anal canal and potential locations of peri-anal abscesses [Reprinted from Szurowska E. Perianal fistulas in Crohn's disease: MRI diagnosis and surgical planning. Abdominal Imaging 2013; 32(6): 705-718. With permission from Springer Verlag]

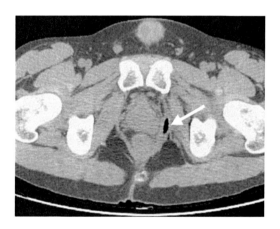

FIG. 17.2 Axial CT scan image of a patient with an air-containing perianal abscess located proximally in the anal canal and not visible on external examination [Reprinted from Szurowska E. Perianal fistulas in Crohn's disease: MRI diagnosis and surgical planning. Abdominal Imaging 2013; 32(6): 705-718. With permission from Springer Verlag]

the abscess. More complex maneuvers are required to effec-tively drain abscesses located proximally in the anal canal.

While drainage of the perianal abscess relieves the acute infection, it does not address the underlying cause of the process. Indeed, about half of all abscesses will result in an epithelialized fistula from the inciting anal gland to the skin overlying the drainage site, a condition known as a **fistula-in-ano**. Patients who develop a fistula will have a persistent sinus track with chronic purulent drainage. Treatment of an anorectal fistula requires eradication of the fistulous tract. A **fistulotomy** is performed by making an incision along the length of the fistula tract in order to fillet it open. This method is effective for most simple fistulas, however, the treatment of complex fistulas can involve a combination of techniques including setons and soft tissue advancement flaps.

In most cases, fistula-in-ano occurs as a consequence of a prior abscess, as described. However, in individuals with **Crohn's disease**, perianal fistulas can develop spontaneously, are often multiple, may occur in unusual locations, and are resistant to therapy. Crohn's disease is a type of inflammatory bowel disease that can affect any site along the gastrointestinal site from the oral cavity to the anus. The most commonly affected area is the small bowel, and the hallmark of Crohn's disease is the development of strictures along the intestines causing bowel obstruction. Perianal involvement is also common among those with Crohn's disease, and is often the clinical manifestation that leads a clinician to suspect the diagnosis.

Perianal fistulae associated with Crohn's disease are notoriously refractory to treatment. In extreme cases, complete fecal diversion with a colostomy may be indicated to allow healing of the perineal area. The recent introduction of **infliximab**—a monoclonal antibody—provides a new treatment option for patients who do not respond to conventional therapy. The use of infliximab has been shown to result in significant clinical improvement in patients with fistulizing Crohn's disease.

Another common benign anorectal process is the **anal fissure**. This condition begins when the anal mucosa is torn, and is then unable to heal due to spasm of the exposed internal sphincter muscle. This spasm counteracts the healing process by further pulling apart the edges of the fissure. The site is irritated with each bowel movement, leading to a chronic non-healing condition. Patients with anal fissures complain of

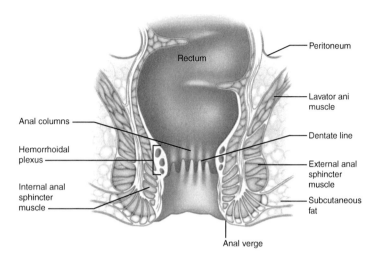

Fig. 17.3 Surgical anatomy for anorectal procedures: rectum, peritoneum, anal columns, dentate line, anal verge, hemorrhoidal plexus,
external anal sphincter muscle, internal anal sphincter muscle, and
levator ani muscle

severe perianal pain and may report some bleeding with bowel
movements.

Since it is the increased tone of the internal sphincter
muscle that interferes with the healing process, treatments for
anal fissure center around creating relaxation of this muscle.
Topical application of **nitroglycerin** induces muscle relaxation, and when combined with a bowel regimen to correct
constipation, may allow for healing of the fissure. **Botulinum
toxin**, injected into the anal sphincter has also been used with
success. Surgical therapy involves a lateral internal **sphincterotomy**, a procedure that divides a portion of the internal anal
sphincter muscle. Each option involves increasing invasiveness and potential complications, but is associated with lower
recurrence rates.

Hemorrhoids are a plexus of vessels located in the submucosal layer of the anal canal (Fig. 17.3). Although hemorrhoids

are present in everyone, the term is usually used to denote the condition when these normal structures become engorged or thrombosed and cause symptoms. The development of symptomatic hemorrhoids is associated with advanced age, pregnancy, or chronic constipation.

Hemorrhoids are classified by whether they are located above or below the dentate line, the point at which the columnar epithelium of anal canal transitions to the squamous epithelium of the anoderm. This anatomic distinction has clinical significance because the innervation of these areas is different. The skin below the dentate line is innervated by somatic nerves, and thus patients with thrombosis of **external hemorrhoids** will experience intense perianal pain. By contrast, **internal hemorrhoids** are generally painless because this area of the body has visceral innervation. Typical symptoms of internal hemorrhoids are bleeding with bowel movements, or prolapse out of the anal canal.

Most hemorrhoid-related complaints can be managed nonoperatively with the use of warm Sitz baths to relieve irritation and stool softeners to decrease straining. Incision and clot enucleation is occasionally used to relive the pain associated with acutely thrombosed external hemorrhoids. In patients who have recurrent symptoms, surgical treatment of the hemorrhoids may be indicated. **Rubber band ligation** is the most widely used technique for symptomatic internal hemorrhoids. In this office-based procedure, the excess tissue is pulled into a device that deploys rubber bands around the base of the hemorrhoid, ligating the blood supply. Surgical excision of the hemorrhoidal tissue — or **hemorrhoidectomy** — can be performed for patients who fail lesser measures.

Surgical Technique

Surgical hemorrhoidectomy can be performed as an outpatient procedure, using either sedation, regional, or general anesthesia as indicated (Fig. 17.4). Patients are placed into jack-knife position and a retractor is inserted into the anal

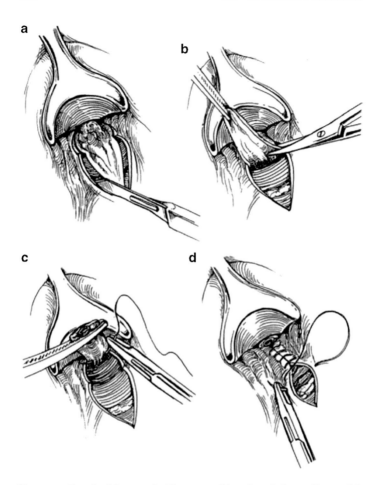

FIG. 17.4 Surgical hemorrhoidectomy. [Reprinted from Singer M. Hemorrhoids. In: Beck DE, Roberts PL, Saclarides TJ, et al. (eds) The ASCRS Textbook of Colon and Rectal Surgery, 2nd edition. New York, NY: Springer Science; 2011: 175-202. With permission from Springer Science]

canal. The hemorrhoidal bundle is grasped and an elliptical incision is made around the column of tissue. Next, the hemorrhoid is carefully dissected out, taking care not to damage the underlying sphincter muscles. Once the main vascular

pedicle is reached, it is ligated and divided. In a closed hemorrhoidectomy the mucosal edges are then sutured together,
whereas in the open technique, the defect is not reapproximated and the wound heals by secondary intention.

In **stapled hemorrhoidopexy**, a specialized circular stapler
device is inserted into the anal canal and advanced above the
dentate line (Fig. 17.5). A purse-string suture is placed
through the hemorrhoidal bundles to pull them into the
device. When the stapler is fired, a ring of rectal mucosa is
excised, resulting in a circumferential ligation of the hemorrhoidal tissue.

Complications

Although hemorrhoidectomy is performed as an outpatient
procedure, it can be associated with significant postoperative
pain. Patients should be provided with narcotic pain medication and stool softeners to reduce straining. Constipation
following hemorrhoidectomy is typically due to opioid use
without proper adherence to a bowel regimen.

Blood per rectum is fairly common after hemorrhoidectomy. This is usually minor, however continued bleeding should
prompt a return to the operating room for examination. Suture
ligation of a bleeding hemorrhoid pedicle may be required.

Urinary retention is also a common occurrence after hemorrhoidectomy, and occasionally patients will require
catheterization for relief. Although typically self-limited, the
inability to urinate should be taken seriously, since it may be
the first sign of a more concerning condition. While rare, the
most serious complication of hemorrhoidectomy or hemorrhoidopexy is **pelvic sepsis**. This condition is presumably
caused by a microperforation of the rectum, which introduces
bacteria into the perirectal space. An ascending infection
ensues with the rapid development of sepsis. Patients typically
present with fever and pelvic pain. If initial treatment with
antibiotics is unsuccessful, operative treatment including
fecal diversion and drainage may be required.

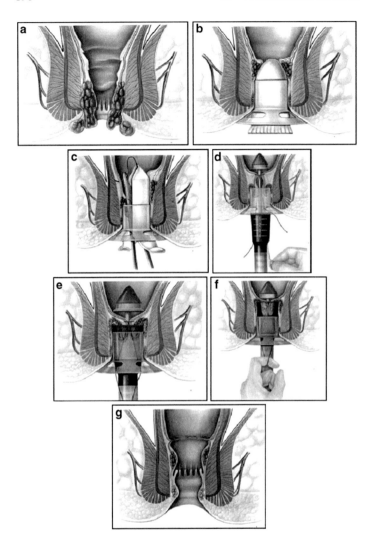

Fig. 17.5 Stapled hemorrhoidopexy. [Reprinted from Singer M. Hemorrhoids. In: Beck DE, Roberts PL, Saclarides TJ, et al. (eds) The ASCRS Textbook of Colon and Rectal Surgery, 2nd edition. New York, NY: Springer Science; 2011: 175-202. With permission from Springer Science]

Classic Case

A 39-year-old man is referred to a colorectal surgeon for a complaint of excruciating anal pain for the past 3 days. The pain is exacerbated by bowel movements and is associated with streaks of red blood on the toilet paper. Examination reveals an elliptical ulceration in the posterior midline, consistent with an anal fissure. The patient is counseled to use warm baths, increase his intake of fiber, and take stool softeners. This initially results in resolution of his symptoms, however after a few months later, following a difficult bowel movement, the pain suddenly returns again. Botulinum toxin is injected into the anal sphincter and results in relief of the pain. The patient experiences occasional mild incontinence to flatus, which resolves after a few weeks. On repeat examination, complete healing of the anal fissure is confirmed. The patient is advised to continue on a high-fiber diet.

OR Questions

1. What characteristics of a perianal fistula should raise the suspicion of Crohn's disease?
   A combination of fissures and fistulae, the presence of multiple fistulae, and fistula recurrence despite appropriate treatment.
2. A 53-year-old male presents with blood per rectum and internal hemorrhoids are visible on anoscopy. Is any further workup necessary?
   Yes, a new complaint of blood per rectum should never be attributed hemorrhoids without performing a colonoscopy to rule out colorectal cancer as a cause.
3. Why can rubber band ligation not be used on external hemorrhoids?
   Hemorrhoids located below the dentate line are innervated by somatic nerves, therefore rubber-banding of external hemorrhoids causes significant pain.

4. A patient with AIDS presents to the emergency room complaining of perianal pain and fever. External inspection of the perineum and digital rectal examination are unrevealing. What test should be ordered next?
   A pelvic CT or MRI should be performed to assess for a possible supralevator abscess.

Anorectal Procedures

Anal fissures
- Laceration of anal mucosa, typically the result of difficult bowel movement
- Underlying anal sphincter muscle is exposed
- Irritation causes spasm of sphincter muscle, which pulls mucosal edges further apart and impedes healing
- Treatment requires inducing relaxation of sphincter muscle
- Topical nitroglycerine causes muscle relaxation
- Botulinum toxin induces muscle paralysis
- Lateral internal sphincterotomy divides a portion of the internal anal sphincter, allowing release of tension

Hemorrhoids
- Spongy plexus of vessels in the submucosa of the anal canal
- Internal hemorrhoids are proximal to the dentate line, have visceral innervation, and present with painless hematochezia or prolapse
- External hemorrhoids are distal to the dentate line, have somatic innervation, and are extremely painful when thrombosed
- Initial management is with increased dietary fiber and stool softeners
- Rubber band ligation used to treat recurrent internal hemorrhoids
- Surgical intervention is reserved for symptomatic, recurrent disease

Perianal abscess

- Arises from obstructed anal crypt gland which is unable to drain normally into the anal canal
- Infected material collects in the soft tissues around the rectum
- Most patients will have a visible abscess on exam; but an abscess high in anal canal will not be apparent on external exam
- Incision and drainage with drain placement relieves the abscess, but not the underlying cause
- About half of cases will result in a chronic fistula-in-ano

Fistula-in-ano

- Most cases are the result of prior perianal abscess
- May arise spontaneously in Crohn's disease
- Fistulae associated with Crohn's disease tend to be multiple, complex, and refractory to treatment
- Fistulotomy to fillet open fistula tract is used to eradicate the process
- In extreme cases, fecal diversion may be indicated
- Infliximab useful in patients with fistulizing Crohn's disease

Technique

- Surgical hemorrhoidectomy: hemorrhoidal tissues are sharply excised; the mucosal defect may be sutured closed or left open
- Stapled hemorrhoidopexy: excision of a circumferential ring of hemorrhoidal tissue using a circular stapling device, which interrupts the vascular channels

Peri-op orders

- Stool softeners
- Oral opioids
- Regular diet
- Ambulatory procedure

Complications

- Bleeding
- Urinary retention
- Pelvic sepsis - rare

Suggested Readings

Vasilevsky CA. Anorectal abscess and fistula. In: Beck DE, Roberts PL, Saclarides TJ, Senagore AJ, Stamos MJ, editors. The ASCRS textbook of colon and rectal surgery. 2nd ed. New York: Springer; 2011.

Kapadia MR, Cromwell JW. Concepts in surgery of the anus, rectum, and pilonidal region. In: Scott-Conner CEH, editor. Chassin's operative strategy in general surgery. 4th ed. New York: Springer Science + Business Media; 2014.

18
Thyroidectomy

Introduction

Most patients undergo thyroidectomy due to the finding of a suspicious **thyroid nodule**, detected either at routine physical exam or upon neck imaging obtained for a separate indication. The finding of a thyroid nodule should prompt evaluation of thyroid function and an assessment for possible malignancy.

Evaluation of a thyroid nodule begins with measurement of serum **thyroid stimulating hormone** (TSH). If the concentration of TSH is low, this suggests negative feedback suppression by a hyperfunctioning adenoma. **Thyroid scintigraphy** can be obtained to confirm the functional status of the nodule. Hyperfunctioning nodules are metabolically active and will demonstrate greater uptake than the background thyroid gland. These so-called "**hot nodules**" are rarely malignant and do not require biopsy. Non-functioning nodules will demonstrate lower metabolic activity than the surrounding thyroid tissue; these **cold nodules** should be biopsied to rule out cancer. If at the outset the concentration of TSH is normal or high, there is no need for scintigraphy; since the concern for a malignancy is greater with a non-functioning nodule, and a fine needle aspiration biopsy will be recommended regardless.

Fine needle aspiration (FNA) is a minor procedure that can be completed in the office with local anesthesia. A high-resolution neck ultrasound is utilized to help target

U. Sarpel, *Surgery: An Introductory Guide*,
DOI 10.1007/978-1-4939-0903-2_18,
© Springer Science+Business Media New York 2014

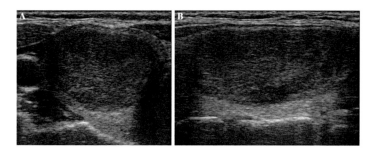

FIG. 18.1 Transverse (a) and longitudinal (b) views from a high-resolution neck ultrasound showing a 3 cm hypoechoic, oval-shaped nodule with well-defined margins in the thyroid; fine needle aspiration biopsy revealed a follicular neoplasm. [Reprinted from Yoon JH. How to Approach Thyroid Nodules with Indeterminate Cytology. Annals of Surgical Oncology 2010; 17(8): 2147-2155. With permission from Springer Verlag]

the lesion and is also useful to assess for other nodules and or enlarged lymph nodes in the region (Fig. 18.1). Results of an FNA can be broadly classified as non-diagnostic, benign, indeterminate, or malignant. Non-diagnostic results indicate that the lesion was not effectively sampled, and repeat biopsy is required. If results of the FNA are suspicious for, or clearly indicative of malignancy, then surgery is recommended. An intermediate designation may indicate a variety of findings, but is frequently used when the lesion is a follicular neoplasm. FNA cannot distinguish between a benign follicular adenoma and a follicular thyroid cancer since an examination of tissue architecture is required, whereas only cytology is obtained by FNA. In these cases, proceedding with a unilateral thyroid lobectomy is generally recommended.

The four histologic classes of thyroid cancer include the papillary, follicular, medullary, and anaplastic types. **Papillary thyroid cancer** is by far the most common subtype and carries an excellent prognosis. In general, lesions less than 1 cm in size can be managed by a unilateral thyroid lobectomy, and a total thyroidectomy is used for larger tumors. Papillary thyroid cancers may spread to the regional lymph nodes, however a neck lymphadenectomy is only indicated if pathologic appearing nodes are encountered.

Follicular thyroid cancer is the second most common type of thyroid cancer. Unlike papillary cancer, follicular thyroid cancer spreads via hematogenous routes, most commonly to the bone or lung. Although specific criteria vary by center, a total thyroidectomy is typically recommended for follicular thyroid cancers since they tend to be more locally invasive.

Radioactive iodine therapy is used following total thyroidectomy for either papillary or follicular cancers in order to destroy any remaining thyroid tissue as well as adjuvant therapy for micro-metastatic disease. Complete ablation of all thyroid tissue allows the use of serum **thyroglobulin** as a tumor marker in surveillance for recurrence.

Medullary thyroid cancer develops from the parafollicular cells of the thyroid that produce calcitonin and are involved in calcium homeostasis. Although medullary thyroid cancer can be sporadic, all patients should be evaluated for multiple endocrine neoplasia syndrome Type II, which is commonly associated with this malignancy. Total thyroidectomy is the recommended treatment since bilateral or multifocal disease is common. **Calcitonin** levels serve as a tumor marker and can be used for surveillance of recurrence.

In sharp contrast to the other thyroid tumors, **anaplastic thyroid cancer** is a very aggressive malignancy whose survival is generally measured in months. Many individuals with anaplastic tumors will have either a prior history of—or a synchronous finding of—a papillary or follicular thyroid cancer, suggesting that these aggressive tumors may arise from a well-differentiated lesion. Patients with anaplastic cancer typically present with a rapidly enlarging neck mass. Regional or distant metastases are present at the time of initial diagnosis in the vast majority of cases, making surgical resection not beneficial. Systemic chemotherapy and/or radiation therapy may be utilized, although their ability to impact survival is limited.

Benign etiologies may also require thyroidectomy. **Toxic multinodular goiter** refers to a gland with multiple hot nodules causing clinical hyperthyroidism. Radioactive iodine ablation is usually the first line of treatment, although surgery is appropriate for patients with large goiters causing airway compression, in patients who require rapid correction of hyperthyroidism, or in those whom radiation is contraindicated. For patients with toxic multinodular goiter, a total or near-total thyroidectomy should be performed. In these patients, surgical manipulation of the thyroid gland can precipitate sudden thyrotoxicosis with tachycardia, cardiac arrhythmia, fever, and agitation, known as **thyroid storm**. Patients with clinical hyperthyroidism should have their thyroid function normalized with antithyroid medications, beta-blockade, and oral iodine as indicated prior to surgery.

Surgical Technique

Most thyroid surgery is currently performed in the standard open manner via a collar incision. New approaches to thyroidectomy, such as endoscopic transaxillary resection are being increasingly performed at specialized centers.

Once general anesthesia is established, laryngoscopy should be considered to assess preoperative vocal cord function. This is especially important in patients who present with hoarseness or clinical suspicion of recurrent laryngeal nerve involvement. Laryngoscopy is also recommended in patients undergoing completion thyroidectomy to confirm that the recurrent laryngeal nerve of the previous operative site is intact.

The patient is positioned with a roll under the shoulders in order to hyperextend the neck. A transverse incision is made along a skin crease in the lower neck and carried down through the platysma muscle. Superior and inferior skin flaps are created by dissecting along the avascular plane beneath the platysma. This exposes the underlying strap muscles, which are spread along the midline to reveal the thyroid gland (Figs. 18.2 and 18.3).

Mobilization of the thyroid lobe is begun by identifying and dividing the **middle thyroid vein** at the lateral aspect of

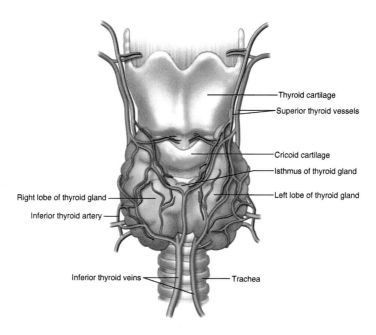

FIG. 18.2 Anterior view of thyroid anatomy. [Reprinted from Porter S, Schwartz A, DeMaria S, et al. Thyroid, Parathyroid, and Parotid Surgery. In: Levine AI, Govindaraj S, DeMaria S (eds). Anesthesiology and Otolaryngology. New York, NY: Springer Science; 2013: 217–240. With permission from Springer Science]

the gland. Gentle downward traction is placed on the gland allowing visualization of the superior pole. The **superior thyroid artery** and vein are ligated en masse, close to the thyroid gland to avoid injury to the **superior laryngeal nerve**. The division of these vessels releases the thyroid gland, allowing for medial rotation of the lobe. Next, the **recurrent laryngeal nerve** is identified and followed along its length. The nerve may lie very close to the inferior thyroid artery, and may even course between branches of the artery. Therefore, no structure in this region should be ligated until the nerve is clearly identified and protected. A nerve stimulator is used by some

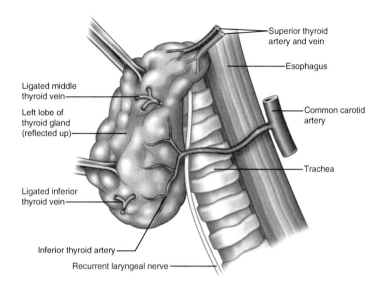

FIG. 18.3 Surgical anatomy during thyroidectomy: trachea, esophagus, common carotid artery, superior thyroid artery, superior thyroid vein, middle thyroid vein, inferior thyroid artery, inferior thyroid vein, and recurrent laryngeal nerve

surgeons to assist in identification of the nerve and verification of its integrity.

Throughout the mobilization of the thyroid, the parathyroid glands are identified and carefully preserved. This is best accomplished by maintaining the dissection as close as possible to the thyroid capsule. The lobe of the thyroid is then further rolled medially until the isthmus is reached. If only a lobectomy is being performed, the thyroid gland is divided at the isthmus. The underlying attachments of the thyroid lobe to the trachea are detached, thereby freeing the specimen. If a total thyroidectomy is being performed, the contralateral lobe is dissected in the same fashion.

Following removal of the gland, the area is irrigated and hemostasis is confirmed. The strap muscles are brought back to their midline position and the platysma is reapproximated. This skin is closed with or without placement of a drain, based on surgeon preference. After total thyroidectomy, thyroid replacement therapy must be initiated to prevent hypothyroidism.

Complications

Nerve injury is the most infamous complication of thyroidectomy, and both the superior laryngeal nerve and recurrent laryngeal nerve are vulnerable during surgery. The superior laryngeal nerve innervates the cricothyroid muscle and injury affects the quality of the voice including pitch change, difficulty speaking loudly, and inability to sing high notes. Although some patients may not even notice the effects of a **superior laryngeal nerve injury**, it is particularly important to discuss this risk with individuals who use their voice professionally.

Permanent **recurrent laryngeal nerve injury** due to inadvertent transection of the nerve is rare in experienced hands. However, transient paresis of the nerve is not uncommon, and is usually due to excessive traction placed on the nerve during dissection. This is especially common following thyroidectomy performed for a large goiter, or in a patient whose tumor lies in close proximity to the nerve.

Patients with unilateral recurrent laryngeal nerve injury will present with hoarseness of the voice, which occurs as a result of **vocal cord paralysis** in a paramedian—or partially open—position. It is important to remember that hoarseness is common following any endotracheal intubation, and therefore no presumption of permanent nerve injury should be made in the immediate postoperative period. If hoarseness persists, laryngoscopy can be used to assess if the vocal cord is indeed paralyzed. Traction injuries to the nerve will demonstrate gradual improvement without intervention. However, if the vocal cord remains paralyzed several months following surgery, return of function is unlikely. Patients with unilateral vocal cord paralysis who have significant symptoms may benefit from procedures to fix the vocal cord in a medialized position.

Bilateral recurrent laryngeal nerve injury can occur in patients undergoing total thyroidectomy, or in those having completion thyroidectomy following a prior ipsilateral nerve injury. Bilateral nerve injury can be devastating, since the vocal cords are paralyzed, causing airway obstruction. Bilateral vocal cord paralysis is typically recognized immediately upon extubation when the patient displays severe stridor. If reintubation cannot be achieved, an emergent tracheostomy may be necessary to restore patency of the airway. Procedures to fix the cords in an open position can relieve airway obstruction but do not restore normal phonation.

Meticulous hemostasis is required during thyroidectomy since even a small postoperative **neck hematoma** can be serious if it causes compression of the trachea. In patients with evidence of airway compromise, the incision should be reopened without delay—at the bedside if necessary—to release the hematoma and relieve hypoxia.

Hypocalcemia as a result of hypoparathyroidism is fairly common following thyroidectomy. In most cases, it is transient and resolves within weeks of surgery. The section on parathyroidectomy details the signs of hypocalcemia and its treatment.

Classic Case

A 38-year-old woman was found to have a thyroid nodule on physical exam by her primary care provider. Neck ultrasound demonstrates a 1.5 cm nodule, and a fine needle aspirate is consistent with a follicular neoplasm. A unilateral thyroid lobectomy is performed and the frozen section evaluation demonstrates that the lesion is a follicular carcinoma. The surgeon proceeds with a completion thyroidectomy, using an intraoperative nerve stimulator to confirm function of both recurrent laryngeal nerves.

At her postoperative appointment, the patient complains of a hoarse voice. This improves over the next few weeks without intervention. She undergoes radioactive iodine ablation without incident, and is started on levothyroxine for thyroid hormone replacement therapy.

OR Questions

1. Which antithyroid medications are commonly in use and what is their mechanism?
   Methimazole and propylthiouracil are the most commonly used antithyroid medications. Both agents inhibit the synthesis of thyroid hormone in the thyroid gland by blocking conversion of iodide to iodine.
2. What medication is used for thyroid replacement therapy?
   Levothyroxine is an oral formulation of T3 which is used to restore a euthyroid state.
3. Is radioactive iodine therapy an option for patients with medullary thyroid cancer?
   No, since these tumors originate from the parafollicular C cells they are not responsive to iodine-based therapies.
4. What is the pyramidal lobe?
   An appendage of thyroid tissue extending superiorly from the thyroid isthmus, it is a commonly found normal variant of thyroid anatomy.
5. What environmental risk is associated with the development of thyroid cancer?
   Radiation exposure.

Thyroidectomy

Thyroid nodule
- Often found incidentally at physical exam
- If TSH is low, obtain thyroid scintigraphy: hot nodules can be observed, cold nodules should be biopsied with FNA
- If TSH is normal or high, proceed to fine needle aspiration

Fine needle aspiration (FNA)
- Performed in office with local anesthesia
- High resolution neck ultrasound used to examine nodule characteristics, assess for lymphadenopathy, and helptarget biopsy
- Non-diagnostic: obtained tissue is inadequate to make a diagnosis, or the lesion was missed
- Follicular neoplasm: FNA cannot distinguish between a follicular adenoma and a follicular cancer
- Suspicious/malignant: thyroidectomy indicated to remove lesion

Thyroid cancers
- Papillary: most common, excellent prognosis, unilateral thyroid lobectomy for tumors <1 cm
- Follicular: good prognosis, total thyroidectomy recommended, hematogenous spread more likely
- Medullary: from parafollicular cells, associated with MEN2 syndrome, radioactive iodine not helpful, calcitonin is tumor marker
- Anaplastic: typically present with an enlarging neck mass, extremely poor prognosis, survival in months

Toxic multinodular goiter
- Multiple hyperfunctioning nodules with hyperthyroidism
- Radioactive iodine ablation is first line of treatment
- Thyroidectomy may be indicated if large goiter is causing airway compression, or if radiation is contraindicated
- Pre-op antithyroid medication and beta-blockers as needed to render patient euthyroid

Technique:

- Consider pre-op laryngoscopy to assess vocal cord function
- Collar incision
- Divide platysma muscle and create skin flaps
- Ligate superior pole vessels en masse, close to the thyroid capsule to avoid injuring the superior laryngeal nerve
- Ligate middle thyroid vein, rotate gland medially
- Locate recurrent laryngeal nerve
- Consider intraoperative nerve monitoring
- Ligate inferior thyroid artery
- Divide gland at isthmus for lobectomy

Complications

- Thyroid storm
- Superior laryngeal nerve injury: difficulty speaking loudly and singing high notes
- Recurrent laryngeal nerve injury: unilateral vocal cord paralysis with voice hoarseness, may be transient if due to edema or excessive traction on nerve
- Bilateral recurrent laryngeal nerve injury leads to vocal cord paralysis and airway obstruction, may require tracheostomy
- Neck hematoma: open emergently if causing airway compromise
- Hypocalcemia: usually self-limited

Peri-op orders

- Advance diet as tolerated
- Calcium supplementation
- Thyroid replacement therapy if total thyroidectomy was performed

Suggested Readings

Suliburk JS, Delbridge L. Thyroid nodule. In: Morita SY, Dackiw APB, Zeiger MA, editors. McGraw-Hill manual: endocrine surgery. 1st ed. New York: McGraw-Hill Professional Publishing; 2010.

Barbra S, Miller BS, Gauger PG. Thyroid gland. In: Mulholland MW, Lillemoe KD, Doherty GM, Maier RV, Simeone DM, Upchurch GR, editors. Greenfield's surgery scientific principles and practice. 5th ed. Philadelphia: Lippincott Williams & Wilkins; 2011.

19
Parathyroidectomy

Introduction

The parathyroid glands are responsible for maintaining normal calcium homeostasis, and surgical resection is most often performed for conditions where hyperparathyroidism disrupts this balance. The production of **parathyroid hormone** (PTH) by the **chief cells** of the parathyroid gland leads to a rise in serum calcium levels by three distinct mechanisms: PTH (1) causes bone resorption leading to the release of calcium into the blood; (2) promotes calcium conservation by the kidneys; and (3) increases absorption of calcium by the GI tract via the production of activated vitamin D in the kidneys.

Hyperparathyroidism is classified into primary, secondary, or tertiary according to etiology. **Primary hyperparathyroidism** is due to an overproduction of PTH, typically from an autonomously functioning adenoma that is not responsive to normal feedback mechanisms. Most cases are caused by a single **parathyroid adenoma**, with a minority being due to two adenomas or four-gland hyperplasia (Fig. 19.1).

The symptoms of primary hyperparathyroidism are classically described as "painful bones, renal stones, abdominal groans, and psychic moans" corresponding to the arthralgias, osteoporosis, nephrolithiasis, pancreatitis, peptic ulcers, constipation, fatigue, and depression associated with hypercalcemia. Because these conditions are vague, nonspecific, and common, many individuals do not realize they are experiencing

U. Sarpel, *Surgery: An Introductory Guide*,
DOI 10.1007/978-1-4939-0903-2_19,
© Springer Science+Business Media New York 2014

a 80–85%   b 5%

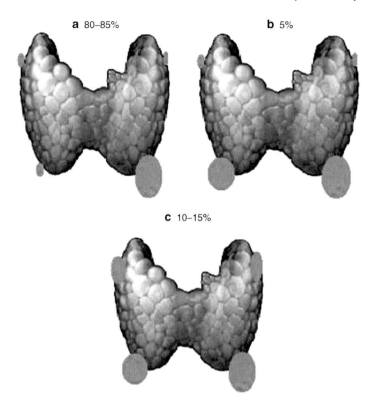

c 10–15%

FIG. 19.1 Parathyroid gland enlargement in primary hyperparathyroidism (**a**) single adenoma, (**b**) double adenoma, and (**c**) multi-
gland hyperplasia [Reprinted from Wu L, Roman S. Conventional
Surgical Management of Primary Hyperparathyroidism. In: Oertli
D, Udelsman R (eds). Surgery of the Thyroid and Parathyroid
Glands. Heidelberg, Germany: Springer Verlag; 2012: 463-473. With
permission from Springer Verlag]

symptoms at all. In fact, it is often only in retrospect that
the signs of hypercalcemia are elicited by a clinician taking a
detailed history.

   The presence of a parathyroid adenoma is diagnosed by
the finding of elevated levels of serum PTH and calcium.

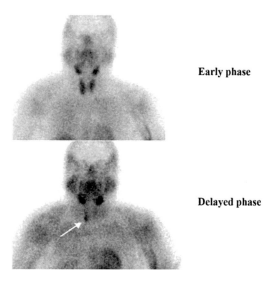

Early phase

Delayed phase

FIG. 19.2 A sestamibi scan of a patient with primary hyperparathyroidism demonstrating an adenoma of the right inferior parathyroid
gland [Reprinted from Gulcelik NE, Bozkurt F, Tezel GG, et al.
Normal parathyroid hormone levels in a diabetic patient with parathyroid adenoma. Endocrine 2009;35 (2):147-50. With permission
from Springer US]

Parathyroidectomy is indicated in all patients who are symptomatic, and also in individuals who are asymptomatic but
display sequelae of hypercalcemia including low bone density
scores, high urinary calcium levels, and decreased creatinine
clearance.

High-resolution ultrasonography of the neck and/or
nuclear scintigraphy (e.g., sestamibi scan) can be used to
identify the location of the parathyroid adenoma (Fig. 19.2).
Preoperative imaging is increasingly being performed to confirm the location of the adenoma, which allows for a targeted,
smaller incision over the enlarged gland. If no localization
studies are performed, an exploration of all four glands is
necessary to rule out multi-gland disease.

Parathyroid carcinoma is a rare malignant tumor of the
parathyroid glands that is another potential cause of primary

hyperparathyroidism. In contrast to patients with a parathyroid adenoma, patients with parathyroid carcinoma typically have symptoms of marked hypercalcemia and may present with hypercalcemic crisis. On physical exam a palpable neck mass may be appreciable. Patients may also present with change in voice due to recurrent laryngeal nerve involvement by the tumor.

Elevated PTH production can also occur in response to low calcium levels, as is seen in chronic kidney disease. In this situation, known as **secondary hyperparathyroidism**, the release of PTH is an appropriate physiologic response to low serum calcium levels, and thus there is no role for parathyroidectomy. The hypocalcemia of renal failure occurs as a result of decreased production of activated Vitamin D by the kidneys. Therefore, renal transplantation is the only cure for secondary hyperparathyroidism caused by kidney failure. It is important to note that patients with secondary hyperparathyroidism do not have the same symptoms as those with primary hyperparathyroidism, since calcium levels are not elevated. Most symptoms of secondary hyperparathyroidism are related to the excessive bone resorption that occurs from the body's efforts to mobilize reserves of calcium and restore normal serum levels.

Tertiary hyperparathyroidism is a condition seen in individuals with long-standing secondary hyperparathyroidism. After years of constant stimulation by low calcium levels, the parathyroid glands ultimately begin to produce PTH autonomously, independent of normal negative feedback. Tertiary hyperparathyroidism persists even after successful kidney transplantation has restored normal renal function. In this setting, PTH overproduction is due to hyperplasia of all four glands and surgical treatment requires a subtotal parathyroidectomy.

Familial hypercalcemic hypocalciuria is an inherited condition that can mimic hyperparathyroidism. Individuals with this diagnosis are usually discovered to have mild hypercalcemia on routine blood tests, but are asymptomatic. In contrast to true hyperparathyroidism, individuals with familial hypercalcemic hypocalciuria have normal PTH levels and paradoxically low urinary calcium levels. The disorder is due to a defect in the receptor that detects the presence of calcium. The parathyroid glands in these individuals are normal, and therefore parathyroidectomy is not indicated.

Human embryology plays a role in the surgical planning for parathyroidectomy. The vast majority of people have four parathyroid glands, although either fewer or greater glands are also possible. The superior parathyroids originate from the fourth branchial pouch. The inferior parathyroid glands are derived from the third branchial pouch and descend past the upper glands en route to their final destination. The inferior glands have a more variable location due to the greater distance traveled. **Ectopic glands** may be located in the carotid sheath, within the thyroid or the thymus gland, in the retroesophageal space, or—rarely—in the mediastinum. The location of ectopic glands becomes relevant when the presence of an adenoma is suspected by biochemical tests, but is not able to be found during a neck exploration.

Surgical Technique

The conventional approach to parathyroidectomy involves a neck exploration with visualization of all four glands (Figs. 19.3 and 19.4). The patient is positioned with the neck hyperextended to optimize exposure. A transverse cervical incision is made and carried down through the platysma muscle. Skin flaps are created and the underlying strap muscles are spread along the midline to reveal the thyroid gland. The thyroid gland is rotated medially and the inferior thyroid artery and recurrent laryngeal nerve are identified as landmarks. All four glands are sequentially visualized and inspected. Once the adenomatous gland has been identified, it is dissected free of surrounding tissues. The vascular pedicle to the gland is clipped and divided, and the specimen is passed off the field. In patients undergoing resection of a parathyroid carcinoma, the malignant gland is removed en bloc with the adjacent thyroid lobe and all regional lymph nodes.

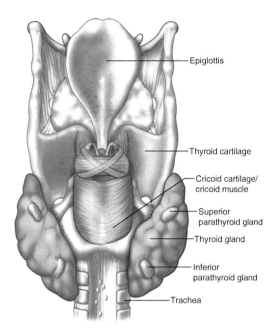

Fig. 19.3 Posterior view of parathyroid anatomy [Reprinted from Gulcelik NE, Bozkurt F, Tezel GG, et al. Normal parathyroid hormone levels in a diabetic patient with parathyroid adenoma. Endocrine 2009; 35 (2): 147-150. With permission from Springer US]

In patients with four-gland hyperplasia, the goal is to resect the majority of the parathyroid glands but preserve enough functioning tissue to allow normal calcium homeostasis. Two options that achieve this are either a 3½ gland excision, or a total parathyroidectomy with re-implantation of a small amount of parathyroid tissue into the sternocleidomastoid muscle or the subcutaneous tissue of the forearm. Cryopreservation of parathyroid tissue is sometimes performed in case the transplanted tissue is found to be insufficient to maintain calcium levels.

Minimally invasive parathyroidectomy utilizes a smaller incision centered over the adenomatous gland, as identified by preoperative localization studies. This approach is associated

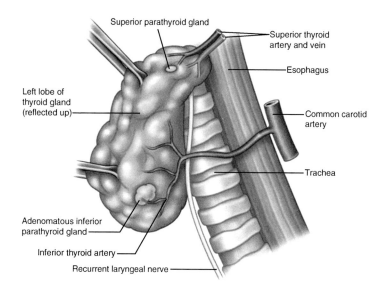

FIG. 19.4 Surgical anatomy during parathyroidectomy: trachea, esophagus, common carotid artery, superior thyroid artery, superior thyroid vein, inferior thyroid artery, recurrent laryngeal nerve, superior parathyroid gland, and inferior parathyroid gland

with shorter operative times. In addition, the limited dissection results in a lower incidence of recurrent laryngeal nerve injury. Since only the target gland is visualized in minimally invasive parathyroidectomy, **intraoperative PTH monitoring** must be used to confirm that no other functioning adenomas remain. PTH levels must drop by at least 50 % within 10 min following removal of the adenoma. If post-resection PTH levels remain high, the surgeon must proceed with exploration of the remaining glands.

Complications

Parathyroidectomy is generally well tolerated and is associated with a low level of morbidity. A neck hematoma is unusual after parathyroidectomy, especially if a minimally invasive approach was used. Transient paresis of the recurrent laryngeal nerve can occur due to stretching of the nerve during surgery and postoperative edema, however permanent nerve damage is rare following parathyroidectomy.

Temporary **hypocalcemia** is the most common complication of parathyroidectomy and is seen in up to 25 % of patients. **Chvostek's sign** is a spasm of the facial muscles caused by tapping the facial nerve. **Trousseau's sign** is carpal spasm elicited by transient occlusion of the brachial artery, as produced by inflation of a blood pressure cuff. These signs as well as perioral numbness and generalized muscle weakness are indications of hypocalcemia. Patients are typically discharged with oral calcium supplementation as a precaution. In most cases the hypocalcemia is mild and resolves in about 1 week. In some individuals, however, postoperative hypocalcemia is severe and prolonged—a phenomenon known as **hungry bone syndrome**. This most often occurs in patients whose hyperparathyroidism was associated with bone disease.

Classic Case

A 56-year-old woman is found to have a serum calcium level of 11.2 mg/dL on routine lab tests obtained by her primary care physician. On follow-up, a PTH level is found to be elevated, as are 24-h urine calcium levels. A high-resolution ultrasound of the neck is performed and suggests the presence of an adenoma of the left inferior parathyroid gland. A sestamibi scan shows increased uptake only at that same site, confirming the presence of a single parathyroid adenoma.

The patient undergoes an uneventful minimally invasive parathyroidectomy. Upon resection of the adenomatous gland, the intraoperative PTH level drops to less than 50 % of the preoperative value. She is discharged home on oral calcium supplements. On the morning following surgery she calls her surgeon's office with a complaint of perioral numbness. The dose of calcium supplements is increased which leads to resolution of the symptoms. At her postoperative visit, 1 week later, serum calcium levels are normal.

OR Questions

1. What is the most common cause of hypercalcemia in outpatients?
   A parathyroid adenoma.
2. What is the most common cause of hypercalcemia in hospitalized patients?
   Bony metastases from a malignancy.
3. An otherwise healthy woman is found to have mild hypercalcemia on routine labs. Her PTH level is normal, and 24-h urine calcium levels are low. A neck ultrasound is performed, but fails to identify an adenoma, why?
   This patient likely has familial hypercalcemic hypocalciuria, which is not associated with a parathyroid adenoma.
4. Individuals diagnosed with parathyroid hyperplasia should be screened for which endocrine syndromes?
   Hyperparathyroidism is associated with multiple endocrine neoplasia type I and type IIa.
5. What is calciphylaxis?
   Calciphylaxis is a poorly understood condition seen in patients with end-stage renal disease, where calcification of the arterioles leads to severe skin necrosis. Many patients with calciphylaxis have elevated PTH levels, and urgent parathyroidectomy may be recommended in patients who are unresponsive to medical therapy.

Parathyroidectomy

Hyperparathyroidism

- Primary: hypersecretion of parathyroid hormone (e.g. by an adenoma or carcinoma), leading to hypercalcemia
- Secondary: chronic renal insufficiency causes hypocalcemia, which appropriately stimulates PTH secretion to attempt to normalize calcium levels
- Tertiary: autonomous gland hyperfunction develops in patients with long-standing secondary hyperparathyroidism, parathyroids no longer respond to calcium feedback inhibition, leading to hypercalcemia

Symptoms

- Hypercalcemia leads to "painful bones, kidney stones, abdominal groans, psychic moans"
- The presence of symptoms may not be recognized until after the diagnosis

Embryology

- The superior parathyroids originate from the 4th branchial pouch, but inferiors are from the 3rd pouch and travel a further distance to reach their final location
- The inferior glands have a more variable location
- Ectopic parathyroids may be located in the carotid sheath, within the thyroid or thymus gland, in the retroesophageal space, or mediastinum

Parathyroid carcinoma

- Rare, malignant tumor
- Marked hypercalcemia
- Patients may have a palpable neck mass or evidence of recurrent laryngeal nerve involvement

Imaging
- Preoperative localization of the adenomatous gland allows for a smaller incision
- Nuclear scintigraphy and/or ultrasound are useful modalities

Peri-op orders
- Regular diet as tolerated
- Ambulatory surgery
- Calcium level monitoring
- Calcium supplements

Technique
- Standard: bilateral neck dissection with 4-gland exploration, identification of inferior thyroid artery and recurrent laryngeal nerve, localization and excision of adenomatous gland
- Minimally invasive: pre-operative localization, targeted incision, intraoperative plasma parathyroid hormone monitoring to confirm removal of all adenomatous tissue
- Hyperplasia: either 3 ½ gland excision, or total parathyroidectomy with autotransplantation of parathyroid tissue

Complications
- Transient hypocalcemia
- Hungry bone syndrome
- Neck hematoma
- Recurrent laryngeal nerve injury

Suggested Reading

Sneider MS, Solorzano CC, Lew JI. Primary hyperparathyroidism. In: Morita SY, Dackiw APB, Zeiger MA, editors. McGraw-Hill manual: endocrine surgery. 1st ed. New York: McGraw-Hill Professional Publishing; 2010.

20
Adrenalectomy

Introduction

The adrenal glands, although small in size, can be the site of several different types of neoplasms. Primary tumors of the adrenal gland can be either benign or malignant, and the gland is also a common site of metastatic disease from other organs. These neoplasms are the main indication for adrenalectomy.

The adrenal gland is composed of distinct tissue layers, each of which produces a specific hormone. Some tumors of the adrenal gland—known as functional tumors—retain this ability to synthesize hormones, and are characterized by the clinical symptoms caused by this hormone overproduction. An **aldosteronoma** is a tumor of the adrenal cortex that causes an excess release of the hormone aldosterone. Most patients with this pathology present with poorly controlled high blood pressure despite therapy with multiple antihypertensives. These tumors are typically benign, but resection is indicated for treatment of the hypertension.

Cortisol overproduction, as caused by **cortisol-producing adenomas** of the adrenal cortex can lead to the development of **Cushing's syndrome**. This syndrome can also occur by any upstream cause of increased cortisol production, including adrenocorticotropic hormone (ACTH) producing tumors of the pituitary or other ectopic site. Iatrogenic Cushing's syndrome can be seen in patients who are prescribed long-term steroid therapy. The hallmarks of this condition are central

U. Sarpel, *Surgery: An Introductory Guide*,
DOI 10.1007/978-1-4939-0903-2_20,
© Springer Science+Business Media New York 2014

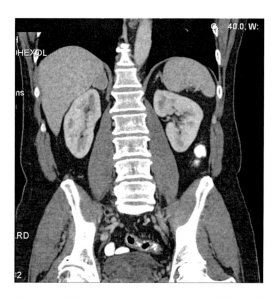

FIG. 20.1 Coronal CT scan image of a patient with a right adrenal pheochromocytoma; note the normal adrenal gland on the left

obesity with purple striae, hirsutism, hypertension, and hyperglycemia. Patients undergoing resection of a cortisol-producing adenoma must be started on a steroid taper post-operatively in order to allow the suppressed contralateral gland to resume normal steroid production.

In addition to the mineralocorticoids and the glucocorticoids discussed above, the adrenal cortex also produces the sex steroids. Androgen and estrogen secreting tumors of the adrenal gland do exist, however these are extremely rare.

Pheochromocytomas are tumors of the adrenal medulla that produce an overabundance of catecholamines (Fig. 20.1). As expected, surges of catecholamine release from these tumors cause symptoms including intense perspiration, palpitations, and tremor. While these symptoms are episodic, many patients also have sustained hypertension—often unresponsive to medical management. Catecholamine release by these tumors may be spontaneous, or can be induced by events such as strenuous physical exertion, trauma, and ingestion of tyramine-rich foods.

The diagnosis of a pheochromocytoma is made by a combination of imaging appearance and the results of urine and serum tests for catecholamine products. No attempt at biopsy should be made since the procedure can initiate a catecholamine release. Nuclear scintigraphy (i.e., MIBG or PET scan) can be used to detect occult or metastatic lesions in cases where no mass is apparent on imaging but is suggested by biochemical data.

The majority of pheochromocytomas are benign in that they do not have the ability to metastasize, however the clinical symptoms produced can be severe and warrant resection. Importantly, anesthetic induction and manipulation of the tumor are strong stimulants for catecholamine release. Therefore any patient undergoing resection of a pheochromocytoma must undergo alpha and then beta-adrenergic blockage to prevent a hypertensive crisis at surgery.

Given the increased use of imaging tests in medicine, it is not uncommon to discover small adrenal lesions in an asymptomatic patient on imaging obtained for other reasons. These lesions, which have been coined **incidentalomas**, present a therapeutic challenge for the physician. Nondiscretionary removal of every adrenal lesion would lead to many unnecessary operations since a significant number of these lesions would remain small and clinically insignificant. Exact criteria vary, however adrenalectomy is generally recommended for any tumor found to be hormone producing, or for lesions whose size exceeds 3–5 cm, since increasing size correlates with malignancy.

Adrenocortical carcinoma is a rare, aggressive malignancy of the adrenal gland that can arise de novo, or as a result of malignant transformation of any of the adenomas described above. Patients with functioning tumors may present with the symptoms associated with that hormone. However nonfunctional tumors are typically not discovered until the enlarging size of the mass causes symptoms such as back pain due to local invasion. Unfortunately, most patients already have metastases at the time of diagnosis.

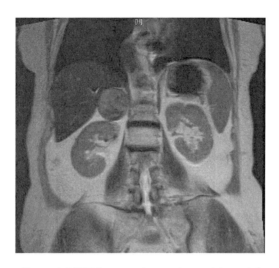

FIG. 20.2 Coronal MRI image of a patient with a right adrenal metastasis from hepatocellular carcinoma

Adrenal metastases can be seen in patients with primary tumors of other organs, including the breast, lung, kidney, liver, and in patients with melanoma and lymphoma (Fig. 20.2). Adrenalectomy is occasionally indicated in select patients with an isolated adrenal metastasis and well-controlled disease.

Surgical Technique

There are multiple surgical approaches for performing an adrenalectomy, including transabdominal and posterior retroperitoneal, both of which may be performed laparoscopic or open. The laparoscopic posterior retroperitoneal approach has several notable advantages and has largely become the standard of care, particularly for small, benign lesions. The open transabdominal approach is more commonly used for larger malignancies, when the tumor is locally invasive, or in situations where vascular control of the vena cava is necessary. Other techniques such as the open retroperitoneal

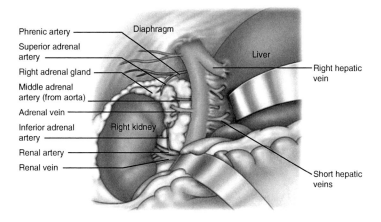

Phrenic artery

Superior adrenal
artery

Right adrenal gland

Middle adrenal
artery (from aorta)

Adrenal vein

Inferior adrenal
artery

Renal artery

Renal vein

Diaphragm

Liver

Right kidney

Right hepatic
vein

Short hepatic
veins

FIG. 20.3 Surgical anatomy during a right open adrenalectomy: inferior vena cava, short hepatic veins, renal vein, adrenal vein, renal artery, inferior adrenal artery, middle adrenal artery, superior adrenal artery, phrenic artery, and kidney

approach may be indicated in select cases. Each version of adrenalectomy must be modified slightly to accommodate the differing venous anatomy of the right and left glands.

An **open adrenalectomy** is performed with either a midline or subcostal incision. The major disadvantage of this approach is that in order to reach the adrenal glands, the surgeon must mobilize all of the intervening intrabdominal organs. To approach the right adrenal gland, the hepatic flexure of the colon is first dissected down (Fig. 20.3). Next, the liver must be extensively mobilized and rolled medially until the inferior vena cava is exposed. The right adrenal vein drains directly into the vena cava and care must be taken not to avulse this structure.

The technique for a left adrenalectomy differs in that the splenic flexure of the colon is first mobilized, and the tail of the pancreas as well as the spleen must then be dissected away to expose the gland beneath. The left adrenal vein is longer than on the right side, and drains into the left renal vein (Fig. 20.4). Once the adrenal vein has been ligated and

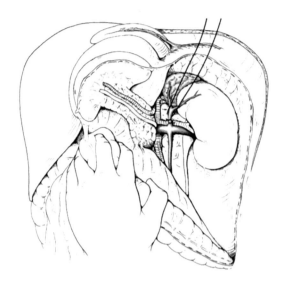

FIG. 20.4 Surgical anatomy during a left open adrenalectomy; note that the left adrenal vein drains into the left renal vein [Reprinted from De Toma G, Polistena A, Cavallaro G. Open Adrenalectomy. In: Valeri A, Bergamini C, Bellantone R, et al (eds). Surgery of the Adrenal Gland. Milan, Italy: Springer Verlag 2013: 145-160. With permission from Springer Verlag]

divided, the dissection is continued along the edge of the gland. Several small arteries provide the blood supply to the adrenal gland, and these vessels are cauterized or clipped and then transected. A laparoscopic transabdominal adrenalectomy essentially mirrors the open approach, but has the advantage of smaller incisions.

By contrast, a **laparoscopic retroperitoneal adrenalectomy** is a completely different technique which uses a posterior approach to the adrenal gland. The major benefit of the retroperitoneal approach is that it provides the most direct access to the gland, without the need to mobilize and risk injury to other organs (Fig. 20.5). The retroperitoneal approach is especially ideal for patients with intraabdominal adhesions from prior abdominal operations. The major disadvantage of the

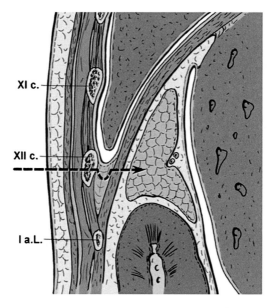

XI c.

XII c.

I a.L.

Fig. 20.5 Posterior approach to the adrenal gland [Reprinted from De Toma G, Polistena A, Cavallaro G. Open Adrenalectomy. In: Valeri A, Bergamini C, Bellantone R, et al (eds). Surgery of the Adrenal Gland. Milan, Italy: Springer Verlag 2013: 145-160. With permission from Springer Verlag]

approach is that the working space is limited, and the different perspective can make it challenging to visualize the anatomy.

A laparoscopic retroperitoneal adrenalectomy can be performed with the patient in either a lateral decubitus or a prone position. An incision is made just below the tip of the 12th rib, the peritoneum is gently swept aside, and a trocar is inserted. A balloon is inserted into retroperitoneum and slowly inflated to create a working space. The adrenal is identified and dissection is carried out circumferentially heading towards the medial aspect of the gland. The adrenal vein is identified and divided using either clips or an energy device. The adrenal gland is placed into a bag and removed from one of the ports, which can be enlarged to accommodate the specimen.

Complications

In general, adrenalectomy is a well-tolerated and safe procedure. Each approach carries the morbidities inherent to the
type of incision used, such as a trocar site hernia or wound
infection. The most common complications of adrenalectomy
are those from damage to other structures caused during the
approach to the adrenal gland, such as injury to the tail of the
pancreas or an inadvertent enterotomy.

The most serious risk of adrenalectomy common to all
approaches is hemorrhage due to avulsion of the adrenal
vein. Vascular control during a right adrenalectomy is particularly challenging because the right adrenal vein is less
than 1 cm in length and empties directly into the inferior
vena cava. Excessive traction on this vessel can easily lead to
a tear that propagates into the vena cava leading to life-
threatening hemorrhage. Bleeding is more difficult to control
from the retroperitoneal approach due to the limited working space and lack of access to the abdomen. Therefore cases
in which there is concern over the ability to obtain vascular
control of the adrenal vein should be performed via the open
approach.

In addition, each type of adrenal tumor has its own potential operative complication associated with its particular hormone. In patients with a cortisol-producing adenoma, normal
cortisol production is suppressed as a result of a negative
feedback loop. Therefore, these patients must be started on a
steroid taper postoperatively in order to allow the suppressed
contralateral gland to resume normal steroid production.
Without supplemental steroids, these patients are at risk for
acute adrenal insufficiency.

Patients with a pheochromocytoma can experience significant hemodynamic lability during adrenalectomy. An **acute
hypertensive crisis** can occur despite appropriate preoperative alpha and beta-adrenergic blockage. Therefore, it is
critical that the anesthesiologist be familiar with the physiology of pheochromocytomas and have available a variety of
vasoactive medications at hand.

Classic Case

A 42-year-old woman with no past medical history is scheduled for an elective laparoscopic cholecystectomy for biliary colic. Upon induction of general anesthesia, she suddenly becomes hypertensive to 205/120 mmHg. The procedure is aborted and the anesthesiologist is able to normalize the blood pressure. The patient is awakened from anesthesia and a full evaluation is initiated.

A CT scan is obtained and demonstrates a 4 cm well-circumscribed right adrenal mass, with no evidence of metastatic disease. 24-h urinary fractionated catecholamines and metanephrines are elevated, confirming the suspicion of a pheochromocytoma. The patient is started on phenoxybenzamine for alpha-adrenergic blockade for a period of 10 days. Propranolol is added for beta-blockade and continued for an additional 2 days. The patient then undergoes a laparoscopic retroperitoneal adrenalectomy without any hemodynamic instability. She is kept under close observation during the postoperative period and has an uneventful recovery.

OR Questions

1. Pheochromocytoma is commonly associated with which familial syndromes?
   Multiple endocrine neoplasia type 2, von Hippel-Lindau's disease.
2. A patient with clinical and biochemical evidence of a pheochromocytoma has no adrenal masses seen on CT. What are the other potential locations of the tumor?
   While 90 % of pheochromocytomas are located in the adrenal gland, extra-adrenal possibilities include the para-aortic sympathetic chain, the organ of Zuckerkandl, and the urinary bladder.
3. What is the most common cause of Cushing's syndrome?
   Exogenous steroid administration.

4. What is Cushing's disease?

   Cushing's disease is when the syndrome is caused by over-production of ACTH by the pituitary gland.

5. What is Conn's syndrome?

   The combination of hypertension and hypokalemia, typically caused by an aldosterone-secreting adenoma.

6. What features of an adrenal mass on imaging suggest malignancy?

   Size greater than 5 cm is the most concerning feature; other imaging characteristics suggesting malignancy include irregular shape, heterogeneous enhancement, and adjacent lymphadenopathy.

7. What panel of tests should be ordered to evaluate whether an incidentaloma is a functioning tumor?

   24-hour urine catecholamines and metanephrines will establish whether the mass is a pheochromocytoma; a dexamethasone suppression test will assess for a cortisol-producing adenoma; measurement of plasma aldosterone, renin, and potassium levels will ascertain if the lesion is an aldosteronoma.

Adrenalectomy

Pheochromocytoma
- Catecholamine secreting tumor
- 90% arise in adrenal gland
- Classic symptoms: hypertension, paroxysmal headache, perspiration, tremor, and palpitations
- Associated with familial syndromes including MEN2 and von Hippel-Lindau
- Diagnostic test is measurement of 24-hour urine catecholamines and metanephrines
- Imaging with CT or MRI usually demonstrates a mass, if not scintigraphy (MIBG or PET) can be considered
- Patients must be prepared for surgery with alpha and then beta-adrenergic blockade to prevent hypertensive crisis

Aldosteronoma
- Conn's syndrome: hypertension and hypokalemia
- Should suspect in a patient with hypertension refractory to medical therapy

Adrenocortical carcinoma
- Most patients have metastases at the time of diagnosis
- Suspect malignancy if tumor >5 cm, has irregular shape, heterogeneous enhancement, or adjacent lymphadenopathy

Cortisol-producing adenoma
- Excess cortisol production causes Cushing's syndrome: truncal obesity, purple striae, moon facies, buffalo hump
- The most common cause of Cushing's syndrome is exogenous glucocorticoid administration
- Cushing's disease is when this syndrome is caused by overproduction of ACTH by the pituitary gland

Incidentaloma

- Adrenal mass discovered incidentally on unrelated imaging
- All hormonally active tumors should be resected
- Nonfunctional tumors >5 cm should be resected since increasing size correlates with malignant transformation

Peri-op orders

- Close hemodynamic monitoring
- Steroid taper for patients having resection of a cortisol-producing adenoma
- Advance diet as tolerated

Technique

- Laparoscopic or open via transabdominal or posterior retroperitoneal approach, as appropriate for the clinical scenario
- Lateral to medial dissection of adrenal gland away from surrounding tissues
- Ligation of adrenal vein
- For pheochromocytomas tumor manipulation should be minimized in order to reduce the risk of sudden catecholamine release

Complications

- Intra-operative hemorrhage due to avulsion of adrenal vein
- Pheochromocytoma: acute hypertensive crisis
- Cortisol-producing adenoma: acute adrenal insufficiency

Suggested Readings

Brunt LM, Rawlings A. Adrenalectomy—open and minimally invasive. In: Fischer JE, Jones DB, Pomposelli FB, Upchurch GR, Klimberg VS, Schwaitzberg SD, Bland KI, editors. Fischer's mastery of surgery. 6th ed. Philadelphia: Lippincott Williams & Wilkins; 2012.

Moalem J, Clark O. Incidentalomas and metastases to the adrenal gland. In: Morita SY, Dackiw APB, Zeiger MA, editors. McGraw-Hill manual: endocrine surgery. 1st ed. New York: McGraw-Hill Professional Publishing; 2010.

21

Breast Surgery

Introduction

A surgeon is often asked to see a patient after the finding of
a palpable breast mass, or because of a concerning finding on
mammography. Although the majority of masses are benign
lesions such as a cyst or **fibroadenoma**, a full evaluation is
always required to rule out a malignancy. Assessment begins
with a detailed history to elicit risk factors for breast cancer.
Patients at higher risk are those who have had prolonged
exposure to estrogens, as occurs with young age of menarche,
late menopause, history of exogenous hormone use, and nulliparity or late pregnancy with first child. A detailed family
history is also important in order to determine whether there
may be a genetic predisposition to the development of breast
cancer. Physical examination includes inspection and palpation of both breasts and the axillae, followed by imaging.

Guidelines for early detection of breast cancer vary, but
generally include a baseline mammogram at 40 or 50 years of
age, followed by **mammography** every 1–2 years. Suspicious
findings may include an area of **microcalcifications** (Fig. 21.1)
or a solid, spiculated mass (Fig. 21.2). The **BI-RADS** classification system uses a scale of 0–5 to rate mammographic findings, with 0 meaning an insufficient exam, 1 describing a
normal exam with no findings, 2 representing benign findings,
3 meaning findings that are probably benign, 4 expressing a
suspicious abnormality, and 5 being highly suggestive of

U. Sarpel, *Surgery: An Introductory Guide*,
DOI 10.1007/978-1-4939-0903-2_21,
© Springer Science+Business Media New York 2014

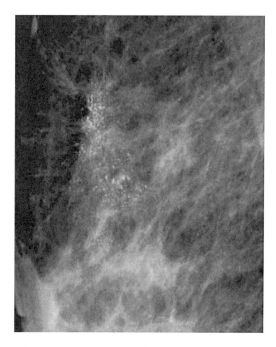

FIG. 21.1 Mammogram demonstrating a focal area of microcalcifications [Reprinted from Obenauer S, Hermann KP, Grabbe E. Applications and literature review of the BI-RADS classification. European Radiology 2005; 15(5): 1027-1036. with permission from Springer Verlag]

malignancy. However, it is important to remember that greater than 10 % of malignant lesions are mammographically occult. Other imaging modalities are also used to assess for breast cancer. Ultrasonography is a useful adjunct in younger patients and for those with breast cysts. **Breast MRI** can be used in select patients, but is overly sensitive and too nonspecific for use as a general screening test.

Patients with concerning findings should undergo biopsy of the site to determine the pathology. If the lesion is easily palpable, a fine needle aspiration or core biopsy can be

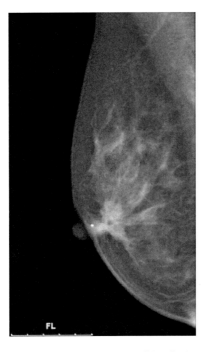

FIG. 21.2 Mammogram demonstrating a solid, spiculated mass behind the nipple that was subsequently confirmed to be invasive breast cancer

performed. For non-palpable masses, imaging-guided biopsies such as a **stereotactic biopsy** can be obtained.

If the biopsy results demonstrate invasive breast cancer, the next step for most patients is formal surgical resection of the tumor. An extensive metastatic work-up is not required in the absence of specific symptoms. Patients with invasive breast cancer have essentially two options for surgical therapy: a **modified radical mastectomy**, or **lumpectomy** with adjuvant **breast radiation**. Large, multicenter studies with long-term follow-up have demonstrated that both approaches result in equivalent overall survival, and therefore treatment decisions should be made on a patient-by-patient basis.

Preoperative chemotherapy is occasionally used for patients with inflammatory breast cancer, or for those with large tumors in whom a reduction in tumor size would allow breast-conserving therapy.

Axillary lymph node staging is an important factor in determining treatment and prognosis in patients with invasive breast cancer. Patients with enlarged palpable nodes in the axilla likely have nodal involvement and should undergo a complete **axillary lymphadenectomy** in conjunction with breast resection. Patients with a clinically negative axilla can undergo a **sentinel lymph node biopsy**, which is associated with a significantly lower risk of **lymphedema**. In the past, if the sentinel node was positive for tumor, patients uniformly underwent completion lymphadenectomy. However, recent findings demonstrate that this procedure may not be necessary in patients with minimal nodal involvement.

Following surgery, decisions regarding adjuvant endocrine therapy and/or systemic chemotherapy are based on the size of the lesion, nodal involvement, the tumor's hormone receptor status, and the patient's age and overall health. In general, most patients except those with the smallest node-negative tumors will be recommended to receive systemic chemotherapy. However, the decision to pursue chemotherapy must always be weighed against the associated toxicities, particularly in older patients with multiple comorbidities.

Most breast cancers retain functional **estrogen and progesterone (ER/PR)**, and this feature can be exploited with hormonal treatments that block these sites. **Tamoxifen** is an agent that acts as an antiestrogen in the breast through competitive binding of the receptor, and is used in premenopausal women. **Anastrazole** is an aromatase inhibitor that blocks aromatase, the enzyme required for final step of estrogen synthesis, and is used in postmenopausal women. The use of antihormonal agents has been shown to decrease recurrence and improve outcomes in patients with ER/PR positive breast cancer.

Targeted therapy for breast cancer represents a recent significant advance in the field. HER2 is a transmembrane receptor whose downstream signaling is involved in cell proliferation. Amplification of the source gene for HER2 occurs in a subset of breast cancers, and is strongly associated with a worse prognosis. **Trastuzumab** is a monoclonal antibody that binds with the receptor and interferes with its function. In patients with HER2-positive breast cancer, trastuzumab therapy has been shown to result in longer survival.

Other than invasive breast cancer, another potential biopsy finding is **ductal carcinoma in situ** (DCIS). This lesion typically manifests on a mammogram as an area of microcalcifications, usually with no corresponding palpable mass. DCIS is considered a precursor to invasive breast cancer, but lacks metastatic potential because the malignant cells have not yet penetrated the basement membrane. Complete excision of the area with a lumpectomy and adjuvant radiation is sufficient treatment, although patients with DCIS involving a large portion of the breast may require a mastectomy to clear all the disease. In pure DCIS, the chance of lymph node metastases is negligible, and therefore lymph node sampling is not generally indicated. However, if the entire breast is diffusely involved with DCIS, a small focus of invasive cancer may escape detection, and sentinel lymph node biopsy can be considered. Tamoxifen may be recommended in select patients with DCIS who are considered to be high risk.

Another entity called **lobular carcinoma in situ** (LCIS) can also be found on breast biopsy. LCIS itself is not associated with any mammographic or physical exam findings, and is only discovered incidentally in the background of a biopsy performed for other reasons. Unlike DCIS, LCIS is not a premalignant lesion, but is considered a marker of high-risk status. Women with LCIS have an approximately 25 % chance of developing breast cancer in their lifetime, and the risk of subsequent cancer is equal in both breasts. Tamoxifen is generally recommended in patients with LCIS to decrease the odds of developing breast cancer.

The vast majority of patients with breast cancer do not have a genetic risk factor for the malignancy. However, genetic screening should be considered for women with breast cancer diagnosed before age 40 years, and those with a family history of two or more relatives with breast cancer or ovarian cancer, or male breast cancer in the family. **BRCA1** and **BRCA2** are the major breast cancer susceptibility genes, and are found in about 5–10 % of women with breast cancer. Importantly, these mutations can be inherited from either maternal or paternal relatives. Patients with a gene mutation have considerable lifetime risk of developing breast cancer—as high as 80 % in some studies. Patients with proven gene mutations should be counseled about the importance of life-long screening. Some BRCA gene mutation carriers may elect to undergo **prophylactic bilateral mastectomy**.

Surgical Technique

The aim of a **mastectomy** is to remove all breast tissue, including the portion that extends into the axilla, known as the **tail of Spence** (Fig. 21.3). A transverse elliptical incision is made in the skin, encompassing the nipple-areolar complex and any prior biopsy site. Electrocautery or sharp dissection is used to separate the breast parenchyma from the overlying skin and subcutaneous fat along an avascular plane. These skin flaps are carried out in all directions, toward the clavicle superiorly, the sternum medially, the rectus sheath inferiorly, and the **latissimus dorsi** muscle laterally. The breast parenchyma is then dissected off the **pectoralis major muscle** beneath. Perforating vessels are carefully ligated and divided.

   If an axillary dissection is part of the procedure (**modified radical mastectomy**), the above dissection is continued en bloc into the axilla. The axillary vein is identified as a landmark and the axillary contents are dissected out, taking care to identify and protect the **long thoracic nerve** and the **thoracodorsal nerve**. This procedure is detailed in the section on lymphadenectomy. Immediate reconstruction of the breast with a tissue flap or implant may be considered for patients with early stage cancer (Fig. 21.4). Alternatively, the skin flap can be closed primarily after placing drains in the surgical bed.

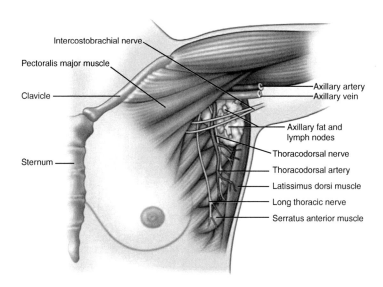

FIG. 21.3 Surgical anatomy during modified radical mastectomy: pectoralis major muscle, latissimus dorsi muscle, serratus anterior muscle, sternum, axillary vein, long thoracic nerve, thoracodorsal nerve, thoracodorsal artery, and intercostobrachial nerves

There are various terms in use for more limited breast resections, including **lumpectomy**, **partial mastectomy**, **quadrantectomy**, and **breast-conserving surgery**. The aim is to remove the area of concern with a margin of normal breast tissue, while still conserving the remainder of the breast parenchyma (Fig. 21.5). For patients whose lesion is not palpable, a localizing wire is placed via imaging guidance prior to bringing the patient to the operating room. A skin incision is made in the region overlying the lesion. If the lesion is centrally located, a curvilinear incision along the periareolar line can be used, and offers the best cosmesis. Electrocautery or sharp dissection is used to divide the breast tissue surrounding the lesion in all directions. The specimen is then carefully oriented with sutures or dye in order to guide further resection if one of the margins is found to be insufficient. Typically the resected tissue is then

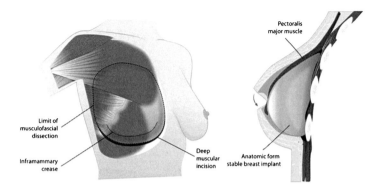

FIG. 21.4 Breast reconstruction using an implant [Reprinted from Rietjens M, Urban C, Sandford M, Kuroda F. One-Stage Breast Reconstruction with Definitive Form-Stable Implants. In: Urban C, Rietjens M (eds). Oncoplastic and Reconstructive Breast Surgery. Milan, Italy: Springer Verlag; 2013:213-226. with permission from Springer Verlag]

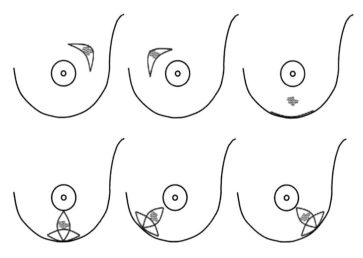

FIG. 21.5 Different skin incisions for breast-sparing surgery depending on the location of the tumor [Reprinted from Blondeel PN, Ali R, Cocquyt V, et al. Current developments in autologous breast reconstruction. European Journal of Plastic Surgery 2005; 28(3): 226-232. with permission from Springer Verlag]

mammogrammed to confirm that the lesion is within the specimen. Once hemostasis is confirmed, the skin is closed. The cavity that is created during a lumpectomy naturally fills with a seroma, allowing the breast to retain its normal contour.

Complications

Both lumpectomy and mastectomy are generally low-risk procedures. The most common complication is a wound infection, which typically presents as cellulitis, and readily responds to antibiotic therapy. Prior breast biopsy is known to raise the chance of post-operative wound infection.

Hematoma formation following mastectomy is unusual, but can occur due to the extensive dissection that is performed. The large potential space that is created, and the compliant skin flaps, can allow the collection of a significant amount of blood. Therefore, attention to hemostasis is essential, particularly if the patient is on aspirin.

The skin flaps that are created during a mastectomy receive their blood supply via perfusing vessels from the underlying layer of subcutaneous fat. **Skin flap necrosis** can occur if this layer is made too thin. It is critical to identify the correct plane between subcutaneous fat and the underlying breast parenchyma to avoid this complication. Necrosis can also occur if the skin is closed with excess tension over an implant, where compression of the perfusing vessels leads to tissue ischemia.

The complications of axillary dissection, notably nerve injury and lymphedema, are discussed in the section on lymphadenectomy.

Classic Case

A 57-year-old woman undergoing routine annual breast mammography is found to have a 2 cm stellate mass in the in the left breast, read as a BI-RADS 4. On history, the patient reports having menarche at age 12 and menopause at age 55. She has never been pregnant, does not take any exogenous hormones, and reports no family history of breast or ovarian cancer. Physical examination of the breast confirms the presence of a hard mass in the upper outer quadrant; there is no lymphadenopathy palpable in the axilla. An FNA of the mass reveals invasive ductal carcinoma.

After consideration of the options, the patient elects to have a lumpectomy with sentinel lymph node biopsy and adjuvant breast irradiation. The sentinel node is negative, and the lumpectomy proceeds uneventfully. On final pathology, the tumor is a 2.1 cm poorly differentiated invasive ductal carcinoma, and is ER/PR positive. The patient undergoes adjuvant breast irradiation, systemic chemotherapy, and is prescribed 5 years of tamoxifen.

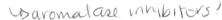 ⟿ aromatase inhibitors?

OR Questions

1. What is the most common solid breast mass found in women younger than age 30?
   Fibroadenoma.
2. In a patient with a palpable breast mass, which should be obtained first—a biopsy or a mammogram?
   A mammogram should be obtained prior to a core biopsy since post-procedure inflammation and scarring may obscure subsequent imaging. Fine needle aspiration prior to imaging is permissible, since the thin needle that is used does not typically disrupt the surrounding parenchyma.
3. A patient is found to have a breast cyst on routine imaging. Following aspiration of the cyst contents, a solid component remains. What is the appropriate management?
   All solid lesions of the breast require tissue sampling for diagnosis. If a breast cyst fails to resolve completely upon aspiration, the residual mass must be evaluated for possible malignancy.
4. What are common sites of distant metastases of breast cancer?
   Bone, lung, liver, and brain.
5. In a patient with invasive breast cancer, what are the reasons to favor selecting a mastectomy over lumpectomy?

Large tumor size, small breast size, multicentric disease, contraindications to adjuvant radiation (e.g., pregnancy), patient preference.

6. A woman with a palpable breast mass undergoes a fine needle aspiration in the office. The subsequent pathology report reveals LCIS. What is the next step?

   A repeat biopsy; LCIS is an incidental finding and does not produce a mass. Therefore, the clinician must conclude that the biopsy missed the actual lesion, and a repeat biopsy is indicated.

Breast Surgery

Benign lesions
- Breast cyst
- Fibroadenoma
- Hamartoma
- Papilloma

Types of breast biopsy
- Fine needle aspiration
- Core needle biopsy
- Ultrasound-guided biopsy
- Stereotactic: mammography-guided biopsy
- Operative: excisional biopsy is performed for a palpable mass, non-palpable masses are localized with pre-operative wire placement

Breast cancer signs
- Palpable mass
- Nipple retraction
- Peau d'orange: dimpled appearance of skin seen in inflammatory breast cancer
- Axillary lymphadenopathy

Breast cancer risk factors
- Age: risk increases with age
- Gender: occurs 100 times more frequently in women than in men
- Early menarche
- Late menopause
- Late age at first birth
- Nulliparity
- Family history
- Personal history

Imaging
- Mammography: guidelines vary, starting age 40-50, every 1-2 years, but about 10% of breast cancers will show no mammographic abnormality
- Ultrasonography: better imaging for young patients or those with dense breasts
- Breast MRI: may be of use in screening high-risk patients, too sensitive for routine use

Ductal carcinoma in situ

- Premalignant lesion
- Clustered microcalcifications on mammography
- Requires excision with clear margins
- Diffuse DCIS may require mastectomy
- If lumpectomy performed, consider postoperative radiation
- In high-risk cases, consider sentinel node biopsy

Lobular carcinoma in situ

- Does not produce a mass or imaging abnormality
- Incidental finding at biopsy
- Considered a marker of high risk for breast cancer, rather than a precursor lesion
- Risk for subsequent breast cancer is equal for both breasts
- Consider tamoxifen

Lumpectomy vs. Mastectomy

- Prospective randomized trials have not demonstrated any survival advantage of mastectomy over lumpectomy plus radiation
- Breast-conserving therapy may not be feasible in patients with a large tumor to breast ratio
- Patient preference and/or desire to avoid radiation therapy are acceptable reasons to perform mastectomy

Adjuvant therapy

- Chemotherapy generally recommended for patients with tumors > 1 cm in size, or with nodal involvement
- Hormonal therapy recommended for patients with estrogen/progesterone receptor positive tumors
- Trastuzumab, an anti-HER2 monoclonal antibody, is recommended for tumors with HER2 protein over-expression

tamotife
aromat
inhib

BRCA 1 and 2 genes
- BRCA gene mutations account for 5-10% of all breast cancers
- Imparts 50-80% lifetime risk of breast cancer
- Carriers are also at increased risk for ovarian cancer
- Consider chemoprevention with tamoxifen
- Consider prophylactic bilateral mastectomy

Technique:
Modified radical mastectomy
- Elliptical incision encompassing nipple complex and biopsy site
- Skin flaps raised
- Breast tissue is dissected off the underlying pectoralis muscle
- Axillary lymph node dissection (see lymphadenectomy section)
- Consider immediate reconstruction with implant or muscle flap

Technique: Lumpectomy
- Also known as partial mastectomy, segmentectomy, quadrantectomy, or wide local excision
- Curvilinear or circumareolar incision made over tumor site
- Excision of tumor with about 1 cm rim of normal breast tissue
- Post-operative breast radiation

Peri-op orders
- Pre-incision antibiotics
- Regular diet
- Drain care
- Arm range of motion exercises for mastectomy

Complications
- Hematoma
- Skin flap necrosis
- Nerve damage or lymphedema if axillary dissection is performed

Suggested Readings

Kwon DS, Kelly CM, Ching CD. Invasive breast cancer. In: Feig BW, editor. The MD Anderson surgical oncology handbook. 5th ed. Philadelphia: Lippincott Williams & Wilkins; 2012.

Gabram SGA. Partial mastectomy. In: Bland KI, Klimberg S, editors. Master techniques in general surgery: breast surgery. 1st ed. Philadelphia: Lippincott Williams & Wilkins; 2011.

22
Lymphadenectomy

Introduction

The differential diagnosis of peripheral lymphadenopathy is long and includes disorders that range from the inconsequential to the rapidly fatal. As a result, surgeons are often called upon to biopsy a lymph node in order to provide the tissue needed to establish the diagnosis (Figs. 22.1 and 22.2).

Lymph nodes can become enlarged for benign reasons such as inflammation, immunosuppression, or in response to a viral or bacterial infection. Features of benign lymph nodes are that they tend to be mobile, tender, have a rubbery consistency, and that—even though enlarged—they retain their elliptical shape. Location is also a useful indicator; for example, the neck is an extremely common site of benign lymphadenopathy, whereas an enlarged supraclavicular node is highly suspicious for malignancy. If a node is of low concern, it may be simply observed for a brief period of time. If the lymphadenopathy regresses, no further evaluation is needed. However, persistent or diffuse lymphadenopathy should be evaluated by biopsy.

Lymph nodes may become involved by a primary malignancy such as lymphoma, or may be infiltrated by metastases from another site. Certain malignancies, such as breast cancer, tend to have an orderly progression through the local lymph nodes before metastasizing to distant organs. However, it is important to realize that other cancers such as most

U. Sarpel, *Surgery: An Introductory Guide*, 245
DOI 10.1007/978-1-4939-0903-2_22,
© Springer Science+Business Media New York 2014

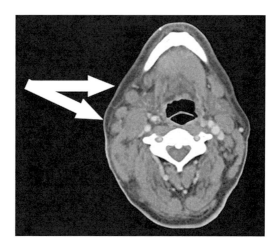

FIG. 22.1 CT scan image of a patient with diffuse cervical lymphadenopathy associated with a non-Hodgkin's lymphoma

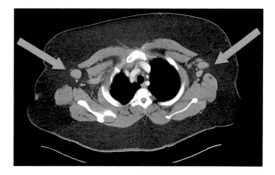

FIG. 22.2 CT scan image of a patient with bilateral axillary lymphadenopathy of unknown etiology for excisional lymph node biopsy

sarcomas, are not associated with nodal involvement, even in advanced stages.

A **sentinel lymph node** refers to the first node that drains a given part of the body. In the setting of cancer, the sentinel lymph node represents the first stop for tumor cells that are in the process of metastasizing from the primary tumor.

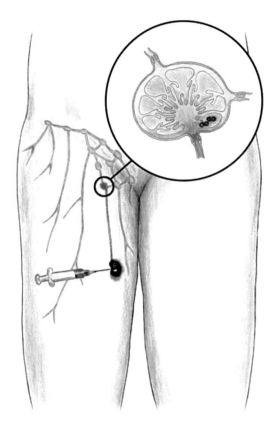

FIG. 22.3 Injection of blue dye into a melanoma lesion in order to identify the sentinel lymph node [Reprinted from Winqvist O, Thörn M. Sentinel Node. In: Schwab M (ed). Encyclopedia of Cancer. Heidelberg, Germany: Springer Verlag; 2009: 2702-2705. With permission from Springer Verlag]

Biopsy of the sentinel node allows physicians to determine whether or not a tumor has begun to metastasize (Fig. 22.3). If there are no tumor cells in the sentinel node, it is unlikely that tumor is present in any of the downstream nodes. While not every tumor type metastasizes in this orderly manner, sentinel lymph node biopsy has proven especially reliable in

breast cancer and melanoma. If the sentinel node is positive
for tumor, a completion lymphadenectomy may be indicated,
but by performing a sentinel biopsy first, most patients can be
spared a full nodal dissection and its accompanying risks.

Surgical Technique

In patients with lymphadenopathy of unknown etiology, an
excisional lymph node biopsy can be performed for tissue
analysis. A small incision is made over the site of lymphadenopathy and the adipose tissue is dissected away to the level
of the node. The target lymph node is placed on traction and
its surrounding attachments are divided. The lymphovascular
pedicle should be isolated and formally ligated, particularly in
large nodes, in order to prevent bleeding or a lymphatic leak.

A **sentinel lymph node biopsy** utilizes scintigraphy and/or
blue dye, to localize the target node in a patient with known
malignancy. In most cases, the site of lymphatic drainage is
intuitive; breast cancers generally drain to the ipsilateral
axilla. However, in cases such as a melanoma located on the
trunk, the sentinel lymph node may be located in the axilla,
groin, or a combination of sites. For sentinel lymph node
biopsy, the primary tumor site is first injected in the nuclear
medicine suite with a radiolabeled substance, typically sulfur
colloid tagged with technetium-99. Images are then obtained
which highlight the location and number of draining nodes.

These images are complemented by the use of vital blue dye;
approximately 3 mL is injected around the tumor site once the
patient is in the operating room. A small incision is made in the
skin over the site identified by preoperative lymphoscintigraphy. The sentinel node is typically identifiable both by its blue
stain and the presence of radioactivity as detected by a gamma
probe. Although referred to as the "sentinel" node, it is not
uncommon for multiple nodes to be identified. Generally, all
nodes that stain blue, or that have >10 % of the radioisotope
counts of the "hottest" node should be excised.

A completion lymphadenectomy, or **regional lymph node
dissection**, may be performed following a positive sentinel

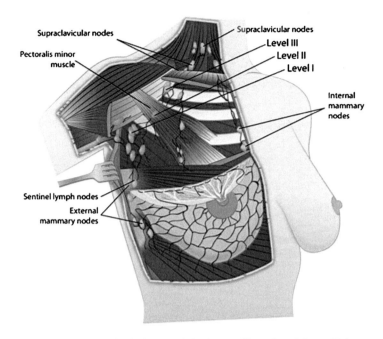

FIG. 22.4 Lymphatic drainage of the breast [Reprinted from Urban C, Rietjens M, Kuroda F, Hurley III J. Oncoplastic and Reconstructive Anatomy of the Breast. In: Urban C, Rietjens M (eds). Oncoplastic and Reconstructive Breast Surgery. Milan, Italy: Springer Verlag; 2013: 13-21. With permission from Springer Verlag]

node biopsy, or for clearly malignant palpable lymphadenopathy depending on the clinical scenario. The most common sites of lymphadenectomy are the axilla and the groin. The specific technique varies by location, but follows similar principles. An incision is made, skin flaps are raised, and the regional lymph nodes are resected en bloc with the surrounding adipose tissue. Intimate knowledge of anatomy is required to prevent inadvertent injury to the blood vessels and nerves at the site.

For an axillary lymphadenectomy, a curvilinear incision is made and carried through the subcutaneous fat (Figs. 21.3 and 22.4). The axillary vein is identified as a landmark and the axillary contents are dissected out, taking care to identify and

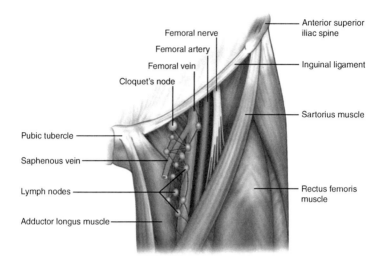

FIG. 22.5 Surgical anatomy during inguinal lymphadenectomy: anterior superior iliac spine, pubic tubercle, inguinal ligament, femoral vein, femoral artery, femoral nerve, saphenous vein, adductor longus muscle, rectus femoris muscle, sartorius muscle, and Cloquet's node

protect the **long thoracic nerve** and the **thoracodorsal nerve**. For an inguinal lymphadenectomy, the borders of dissection are a triangle formed by the **inguinal ligament**, the **sartorius muscle**, and the **adductor longus muscle** (Fig. 22.5). The lymph nodes in this region are dissected free, taking care to identify and protect the femoral vein, artery, and nerve. Generally a drain is left in the resection bed after lymphadenectomy to help prevent a postoperative fluid collection.

Complications

Although technically a clean case, patients undergoing regional lymph node dissection are at significant risk for **wound infection**. Both the axilla and the groin lie within skin folds that are subject to moisture and sweat. Adipose tissue is poorly vascularized, which makes it less resistant to infection. In addition, the extensive dissection during lymphadenectomy results in significant dead space, which permits postoperative collection of fluid and subsequent infection. Finally, the act of lymphadenectomy itself directly promotes infection by interrupting lymphatic drainage, one of the body's natural mechanisms for clearing bacteria. Complete inguinal lymph node dissections are at particularly high risk for wound infection and breakdown.

Lymphedema describes the chronic swelling that occurs in an extremity as a result of lymphatic obstruction, most commonly as a result of lymphadenectomy or radiation. Lymphedema of the arm occurs in about 10–25 % of patients following complete axillary dissection, although in many patients the symptoms are mild and improve with time. Groin dissections are generally associated with higher rates of lymphedema, possibly due to the dependent position of the leg. The chances of developing lymphedema can be lowered with the prophylactic use of compression stockings and rehabilitation exercises. In advanced cases, however, lymphedema can be progressive and debilitating.

Nerve damage is another risk of lymphadenectomy and is of greatest concern during an axillary dissection, due to the number of important motor nerves in the region (Fig. 21.3). The **long thoracic nerve** runs along the lateral chest wall and innervates the **serratus anterior** muscle. Without the tonal contraction of the serratus anterior muscle, the scapula bows outward, creating a deformity known as a **winged scapula**. The **thoracodorsal nerve**, which runs more laterally in the axilla, is also at risk for inadvertent injury. This nerve innervates the **latissimus dorsi** muscle, and its injury causes difficulty with arm adduction. The **intercostobrachial nerves** run transversely across the axilla, and should be spared if possible to avoid numbness in the upper, medial aspect of the arm.

Injury to these nerves can be avoided by a clear understanding of the anatomy of the region. In addition, the anesthesia for an axillary dissection should not include paralysis, so that these nerves can be physically stimulated and their intactness confirmed by muscle contraction.

Classic Case

A 48-year-old woman undergoes a punch biopsy of a pigmented lesion of the mid back and is diagnosed with a 2.0 mm deep melanoma. On physical exam, she has no palpable lymphadenopathy in the bilateral axillary or inguinal areas. A lymphoscintigraphy demonstrates that the sentinel lymph node is located in the left axilla. She then undergoes a sentinel lymph node biopsy and concomitant wide local excision of the primary lesion. Histologic evaluation of the sentinel node reveals the presence of metastases. She subsequently undergoes a completion lymphadenectomy of levels I–III nodes that reveals no additional metastatic nodes. Postoperatively she is instructed to wear a compression stocking, maintain arm elevation whenever possible, and perform range of motion exercises. She is referred to a medical oncologist for consideration of adjuvant therapy.

OR Questions

1. What features make a lymph node's intraoperative appearance suspicious for malignancy?
   Enlarged size, loss of elliptical shape, multiple matted nodes, and—in the context of melanoma—the presence of visible pigmentation in the node (Fig. 22.6).
2. What symptoms at presentation of lymphadenopathy are concerning for the diagnosis of lymphoma?
   Lymphoma is associated with "B symptoms" which include intermittent fevers, drenching night sweats, and unintentional weight loss.
3. What are the sequential lymph node stations in the upper extremity?
   Epitrochlear lymph nodes and axillary lymph nodes.
4. What are the sequential lymph node stations in the lower extremity?
   Popliteal nodes, superficial inguinal nodes, deep inguinal nodes, and external iliac lymph nodes.

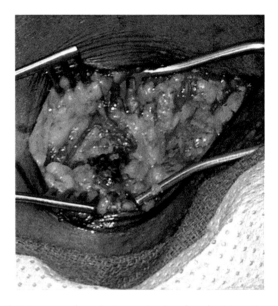

Fig. 22.6 Intraoperative photograph of an inguinal lymph node in a patient with a melanoma of the foot; note the melanin pigment in the node, indicating nodal metastases

5. What is the implication if no sentinel lymph node is visualized after lymphoscintigraphy or injection of blue dye?
   The surgeon must consider the possibility that the lymphatic channels are clogged with tumor, precluding normal drainage.
6. What is the major difference in technique between an axillary dissection for breast cancer versus for melanoma?
   For melanoma all nodes in level I–III of the axilla are dissected, whereas for breast cancer only nodes in levels I and II are taken.
7. For a melanoma in the foot, a preoperative lymphoscintigraphy identifies radioactivity in both the popliteal region and the groin; which site should be biopsied?
   Both sites should be biopsied. This pattern may indicate that the tumor has two separate parallel lymph node drainage

channels, and thus two independent sentinel nodes are present.

8. What is Cloquet's node, and what is its clinical significance?
    Cloquet's node is located just beneath the inguinal ligament, and marks the transition from the deep inguinal lymph nodes to the external iliac nodes. Cloquet's node is typically biopsied during inguinal lymphadenectomy to determine if a pelvic dissection is also necessary.

Lymphadenectomy

Introduction

- Etiology of lymphadenopathy includes infectious, inflammatory, and malignant causes
- Low suspicion for malignancy: tender, mobile nodes, cervical location, recent infection, spontaneous resolution
- High suspicion for malignancy: matted nodes, fever, night sweats, weight loss

Sentinel lymph node biopsy

- Identifies first lymph node draining tumor
- Most commonly used in patients with breast cancer or melanoma
- Recommended for all patients with invasive breast cancer
- Recommended for melanoma ≥ 1mm in depth, or with high-risk features
- Depending on tumor type, patients with metastases to the sentinel node should be considered for completion lymphadenectomy

Technique - Sentinel node biopsy

- Pre-operative injection of radioactive marker into primary lesion, with mapping of drainage pattern
- On-table injection of vital blue dye
- Limited skin incision over target site
- Gamma counter used to localize node
- Identification of nodes that stain blue and/or have high radioactivity
- Pedicle is clipped/ligated
- More than one sentinel node often present
- Residual radiation count must drop to <10% of peak to ensure no additional sentinel nodes remain

Technique - Axillary dissection

- Incision in the non-hair bearing axilla
- Identification of key anatomy including pectoralis major, latissimus dorsi, axillary vein, long thoracic, and thoracodorsal nerves
- Excision of axillary contents
- Placement of drain
- Closure in layers

Technique - Inguinal dissection

- Incision below inguinal ligament
- Identification of key anatomy including adductus longus, vastus lateralis, and sartorius muscles
- Femoral sheath is opened
- Ligation of the saphenous vein at its junction with the femoral vein, and again at distal extent of dissection
- Identification of Cloquet's node
- Excision of inguinal contents
- Coverage of exposed femoral artery and vein with sartorius flap
- Placement of drain
- Closure in layers

Peri-op orders

- Sentinel node biopsy: ambulatory surgery, no drain
- Regional dissection: pre-incision antibiotics, avoid paralytic agents, closed suction drain used, post-op compression dressing, limb elevation
- Regular diet

Complications

- Hematoma, seroma, or lymphocele
- Wound infection
- Lymphedema of the arm occurs in about 1/4th of patients following complete axillary dissection
- Nerve injury to long thoracic nerve causes winged scapula
- Injury to thoracodorsal nerve causes difficulty with arm adduction

Suggested Reading

Neuman HB, Van Zee KJ. Axillary lymph node dissection. In: Kuerer HM, editor. Kuerer's breast surgical oncology. 1st ed. New York: McGraw-Hill Professional Publishing; 2010.

23

Inguinal Hernia Repair

Introduction

An inguinal hernia is a defect in the abdominal wall through which bowel or other abdominal organ protrudes, dragging along with it the peritoneal lining as the hernia sac (Figs. 23.1–23.3). This defect can either be congenital, or it can be an acquired weakness which develops over time.

Indirect inguinal hernias, are congenital hernias caused by the persistence of the **processus vaginalis**. The testicle descends through this tract from the abdomen into the scrotum. This tract normally fuses closed in the third trimester, if it remains patent, however, bowel can herniate out the inguinal canal. In these indirect hernias, the hernia sac is found lateral to the inferior epigastric vessels, along the same path as the spermatic cord—or round ligament in females.

Direct inguinal hernias are acquired hernias caused by increased intra-abdominal pressure and/or weakness of the abdominal wall. Rather than passing through the internal ring and following the course of the spermatic cord, the hernia sac protrudes directly through the anterior abdominal wall, and therefore is found medial to the epigastric vessels. Causes of increased intra-abdominal pressure that lead to hernia formation include chronic cough, pregnancy, ascites, and constipation or prostatic hypertrophy associated with the need to strain. Weight lifting, with its frequent Valsalva maneuvers, can also cause direct hernias.

U. Sarpel, *Surgery: An Introductory Guide*,
DOI 10.1007/978-1-4939-0903-2_23,
© Springer Science+Business Media New York 2014

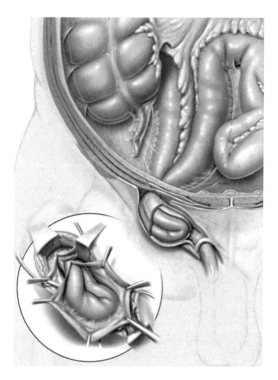

FIG. 23.1 Illustration of a right inguinal hernia containing small bowel [Reprinted from Freundlich RE, Hawes LT, Weldon SA, Brunicardi FC. Laparoscopic repair of an incarcerated right indirect sliding inguinal hernia involving a retroperitoneal ileum. Hernia 2011; 15(2): 225-227. With permission from Springer Verlag]

Although in the past every patient with an inguinal hernia was recommended to have surgical repair, watchful waiting is now an acceptable alternative in individuals who are completely asymptomatic. The most pressing reason to a repair hernia is to avoid the possible complication of incarceration or strangulation. An **incarcerated hernia** is one where bowel becomes trapped within the hernia sac. This often leads to bowel obstruction due to the acute angulation caused at the neck of the hernia defect. Although the bowel is trapped, it still

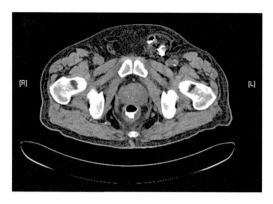

FIG. 23.2 CT scan image of a patient with a left inguinal hernia; bowel with oral contrast is seen within the hernia sac

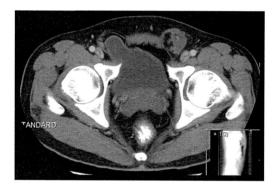

FIG. 23.3 CT scan image of a patient with bilateral inguinal hernias. The right side is a sliding hernia containing bladder wall, the left side contains fluid and omentum

retains a normal blood supply and is viable. However, as edema and congestion develop, the bowel within an incarcerated hernia can become compromised. If the bowel becomes ischemic, this is known as a **strangulated hernia.** Strangulation is a surgical emergency, because if the threatened bowel is not released, gangrene and perforation will develop. Strangulated hernias often present with bowel obstruction accompanied by clinical signs such as fever, tachycardia, and leukocytosis. On physical examination, the site of a strangulated hernia may be erythematous and tender. While an attempt may be made to reduce an incarcerated hernia, a suspected strangulated hernia should never be reduced. Operative exploration is imperative to assess the viability of the bowel and perform resection if indicated.

Surgical Technique

The repair of inguinal hernias has a long, complex history and the various techniques used are the subject of entire textbooks. Similarly the anatomy of the inguinal canal is challenging, and is made more difficult by the many eponyms used to name structures. An intentionally simplified description of the most commonly seen anatomy and techniques are presented here (Fig. 23.4).

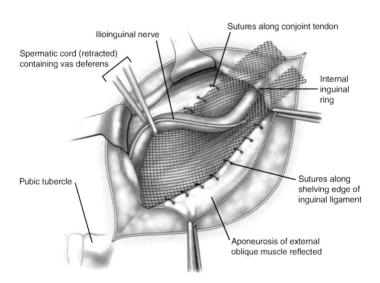

FIG. 23.4 Simplified surgical anatomy during inguinal herniorrhaphy: spermatic cord, vas deferens, ilioinguinal nerve, conjoint tendon, shelving edge, inguinal ligament, mesh, internal ring, and pubic tubercle

For open inguinal herniorrhaphy, an incision is made in the skin above and parallel to the inguinal ligament. This is carried down through Scarpa's fascia. At this level, one or two superficial epigastric veins are often seen, these are ligated. The aponeurosis of external oblique muscle is encountered next; this layer is opened along the line of its fibers and is carried through the external ring, opening it entirely. The underlying **ilioinguinal nerve** should be identified and carefully protected. The spermatic cord is encircled and elevated. If the patient has an indirect hernia, a hernia sac will be seen coming through the internal ring and will lie on the anteriomedial aspect of the cord. This sac may be opened or simply reduced, per surgeon preference. If the patient has a direct hernia, a weak floor of the inguinal canal will be noted, with the hernia bulging up into the field.

Synthetic mesh is now almost universally used to reconstruct the floor and the internal ring. A piece of mesh is cut to size and anchored to **pubic tubercle**. It is then sewn to **conjoint tendon** laterally, and to the **shelving edge** of the **inguinal ligament** medially. A slit is made at the end of the mesh and the two tails are then wrapped around the spermatic cord to recreate a tighter **internal ring**. In females, the round ligament can simply be divided and the mesh laid flat over the entire internal ring. It is important to note that the use of a synthetic mesh is prohibited in the setting of necrotic bowel, or if other sources of infection are present. In these cases, primary repair without mesh should be performed, although the risk of recurrence is likely to be higher. Once the repair is complete, the ilioinguinal nerve is placed back into position, and the layers of the abdominal wall are closed. The strength of the hernia repair comes from the proper placement of the mesh, not in the closure of the subsequent tissue layers.

Unlike other laparoscopic versions of open procedures, **laparoscopic herniorrhaphy** is an entirely different operation than its open counterpart (Fig. 23.5). Both a laparoscopic transabdominal preperitoneal (TAPP) repair and a totally extraperitoneal (TEP) repair are possible. The TEP is the more commonly used technique and will be described here. The TEP repair is done entirely in the preperitoneal space,

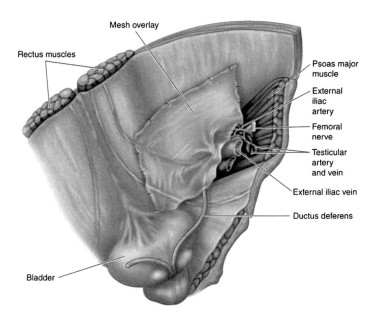

FIG. 23.5 Laparoscopic hernia repair [Reprinted from Straub C, Neumayer L. Abdominal Wall Hernia in the Elderly. Principles and Practice of Geriatric Surgery 2011: 907-925. With permission from Springer New York]

and as a result the anatomy and technique are significantly different than the open approach. First an incision is made below the umbilicus, however only the anterior wall of the rectus sheath is opened. The underlying rectus muscles are retracted to the side and a balloon is inserted into the pre-peritoneal space. The balloon is slowly inflated, thereby dissecting open this potential space. The balloon is then removed and the preperitoneal space is insufflated with gas. If present, the hernia sac of an indirect hernia is reduced. Next, a large mesh is rolled up and inserted through a trocar. It is unfurled, and tacked into place, thereby covering the entire **myopectineal orifice**. Proper tack placement is critical; the surgeon must be very familiar with the anatomy in this region to avoid injuring any nerves or blood vessels. Once the repair is complete, the preperitoneal space is allowed to collapse, and the trocars sites are closed.

The laparoscopic approach is ideally suited to the repair of bilateral hernias since both sides can be easily repaired through the same approach with a single mesh. Laparoscopic herniorrhaphy is also preferred for the repair of **recurrent inguinal hernias**, since this approach takes advantage of fresh tissue planes that were not used in the original operation. In certain patients it is also important to consider that while open inguinal hernia repair can be done under regional anesthesia with sedation, laparoscopic herniorrhaphy requires general anesthesia.

Complications

Although unusual, a **mesh infection** can occur following hernia repair. Like any foreign body, once the mesh becomes contaminated, it must be explanted in order for the infection to resolve. Therefore, synthetic mesh should never be used in a case where contamination is possible, such as in a patient undergoing a bowel resection.

Chronic postoperative pain from **nerve entrapment** can occur if the ilioinguinal nerve is injured in the course of dissection or if the nerve becomes caught in the closure or fixed to the mesh. In order to eliminate the possibility of nerve entrapment, some surgeons intentionally sacrifice the ilioinguinal nerve. This results in numbness of inner thigh and lateral scrotum/labia, but is well tolerated and typically resolves in 6 months.

Inadvertent **ligation of the vas deferens** is possible in cases where the anatomy is obscured due to extensive inflammation. While unilateral ligation has no effect on male fertility, this complication should be avoided, particularly in the presence of bilateral hernias where both structures are at risk.

Ischemic orchitis can occur if the blood supply to the testicle is compromised during surgery. Typically this occurs—not as a result of arterial insufficiency—but instead due to disruption of the venous plexus or too tight a mesh wrap. This results in venous congestion and eventual testicular ischemia.

Most cases of ischemic orchitis are self-limited, and orchiectomy is rarely necessary.

Recurrence of an inguinal hernia should also be considered a complication of herniorrhaphy, although fortunately this has become much less common since the introduction of mesh. The major causes of hernia recurrence are poor surgical technique, excessive tissue tension, infection, and early physical activity. Repeat hernia repairs carry a higher risk of recurrence, and a laparoscopic approach should be strongly considered.

Classic Case

A surgeon is called in consultation for a 65-year-old man with an incarcerated right inguinal hernia. The patient reports that he had previously noticed a bulge in his groin after walking for long periods of time, but it normally disappeared upon lying down. Two days ago the patient developed a cold with a persistent cough and noticed that the bulge was more prominent than usual, and did not reduce. Since then the patient has had nausea and vomiting, and has not passed any flatus or bowel movements.

On examination, the patient is afebrile and hemodynamically stable. His abdomen is distended and tympanitic and there is an easily appreciable bulge in the right groin. The site is not tender and there are no overlying skin changes. Gentle, constant pressure over the site allows for reduction of the hernia. The patient is admitted overnight for observation. He has return of bowel function and is discharged home in the morning with plans for elective herniorrhaphy. At surgery, a direct inguinal hernia is found and is repaired using mesh.

OR Questions

1. What structures comprise the spermatic cord?
   Fibers of the cremaster muscle, the vas deferens, the testicular artery, the pampiniform venous plexus, and the genital branch of the genitofemoral nerve.

2. A patient presents to the hospital with fever, tachycardia, and leukocytosis associated with an inguinal hernia. A strangulated hernia is diagnosed and the patient is taken to the operating room. Upon induction of general anesthesia, the hernia spontaneously reduces back into the abdomen. What should be done?

   A laparotomy/laparoscopy must be performed, to identify if the loop of bowel that was previously trapped within the hernia. If the bowel is necrotic, a bowel resection should be performed and the concomitant hernia repair should be performed without mesh.

3. One week after inguinal hernia repair with mesh, a patient presents to the surgeon with reports of fever, and increasing pain at the surgical site. On exam, there is blanching erythema around the incision and a purulent discharge is expressed. What is the treatment?

   The patient should be taken to the operating room for explantation of the mesh and washout, the skin should be left open.

4. A 55-year-old healthy man is seen for evaluation of a small right inguinal hernia that was found by a primary care physician on routine physical examination. The patient denies any symptoms associated with the hernia. Is surgery mandatory?

   No, watchful waiting is an acceptable alternative to surgery provided that the patient is asymptomatic. However, he should be educated on the symptoms of obstruction and strangulation, should it present a problem in the future.

5. A patient who is on anticoagulation for a mechanical heart valve presents with a symptomatic unilateral inguinal hernia. Should the repair be performed open or laparoscopically?

   An open repair may be preferable since it involves less dissection than the laparoscopic approach, and would therefore lessen the risk of hematoma formation in this patient whose anticoagulation cannot be interrupted.

6. A patient reports persistent groin pain following inguinal hernia repair several months ago. On examination, the wound is well healed and no recurrence is detected. The pain is constant and only temporarily relieved by medications. What should be done?

This patient may have entrapment of the ilioinguinal nerve. This pain may respond to steroid injections or medications for neuropathic pain. If the pain persists, however, the site should be re-explored and a neurectomy performed, along with mesh removal and replacement as necessary.

7. What is a pantaloon hernia?

An inguinal hernia that is both direct and indirect. In other words, the hernia sac straddles both sides of the epigastric vessels, like a pair of pants.

Inguinal Hernia Repair

Introduction
- A bulge in the inguinal area associated with discomfort is the most common complaint
- Incarceration: an irreducible hernia, may cause bowel obstruction
- Strangulation: a hernia containing ischemic bowel

Indirect inguinal hernias
- Congenital defect caused by failure of processus vaginalis to fuse
- Hernia sac is found lateral to the inferior epigastric vessels

Direct inguinal hernias
- Acquired defect due to increased intra-abdominal pressure combined with relative weakness of the posterior inguinal wall
- Inciting factors: chronic cough, constipation, prostatic hypertrophy, pregnancy, obesity, heavy lifting,
- Hernia sac is medial to the inferior epigastric vessels

Anatomy
- Inguinal ligament: band running from anterior superior iliac spine to the pubic tubercle, formed by external abdominal oblique aponeurosis
- Conjoint tendon: formed by edges of the transversus abdominis and internal oblique muscles
- Spermatic cord: contains the vas deferens, pampiniform venous plexus, testicular artery, genital branch of the genitofemoral nerve, cremasteric muscle fibers (the round ligament is the analogous structure in females)
- Ilioinguinal nerve: sensory supply to the skin over the pubis and inner thigh, entrapment during repair can cause chronic pain

Other types of hernias
- Sliding: a portion of the hernia sac is comprised of the wall of a viscus (e.g. bladder, colon)
- Pantaloon: has both indirect and direct component with sac straddling the epigastric vessels
- Femoral: bulge is located below inguinal ligament, often misdiagnosed as an inguinal

Types of repair
- Mesh-free repairs (Bassini, Shouldice, McVay) different techniques of primary tissue reapproximation
- Mesh repair (Lichtenstein): repair using synthetic mesh to supplement the fascia, lowest recurrence rate, but mesh is at risk for infection
- Laparoscopic totally extraperitoneal repair (TEP): mesh is placed within the pre-peritoneal space behind the defect, preferred method for bilateral or recurrent hernias

Technique: Laparoscopic totally extraperitoneal (TEP) repair
- Umbilical incision
- Only anterior wall of rectus sheath is incised
- Blunt dissection performed to create a space beneath the rectus muscle
- Insertion and insufflation of dissecting balloon
- Identification of inferior epigastric vessels
- Reduction of hernia sac
- Mesh is inserted through a trocar and unfolded
- Mesh is placed around cord structures and secured, covering the direct, indirect, and femoral spaces

Technique: Open repair
- Skin incision above and parallel to inguinal ligament
- External oblique aponeurosis is opened
- Ilioinguinal nerve is identified
- Contents of inguinal canal are encircled
- Identification of vas deferens
- Reduction of the hernia sac off cord structures
- Mesh repair of internal ring and floor of the inguinal canal

Peri-op orders
- Pre-operative antibiotics are typically given if mesh is being used
- Can be done under sedation with regional anesthesia, or general anesthesia
- Ambulatory procedure
- No heavy lifting for 4-6 weeks

Complications
- Infection: typically requires removal of mesh
- Ischemic orchitis
- Chronic pain: may be related to entrapment of the ilioinguinal nerve
- Recurrence

Suggested Reading

Sherman V, Macho JR, Brunicardi FC. Inguinal hernias. In: Brunicardi
    FC, Andersen DK, Billiar TR, Dunn DL, Hunter JG, Matthews
    JB, Pollock RE, editors. Schwartz's principles of surgery. 9th ed.
    New York: McGraw-Hill Professional Publishing; 2010.

24

Ventral Hernia Repair

Introduction

Ventral hernia is an umbrella term that includes several types of hernias occurring along the anterior abdominal wall. An **umbilical hernia** is a congenital defect of the umbilical fascia that is very common in childhood. The majority of these hernias close spontaneously by 2 years of age and surgical repair is usually not required. An **epigastric hernia** is also along the midline, but the fascial defect is located higher on the abdominal wall. Given this location, omentum and preperitoneal fat are the most common tissues to become incarcerated in an epigastric hernia. A **Spigelian hernia** occurs at the lateral border of the rectus muscle, at or below the **arcuate line** where the posterior rectus sheath is absent (Fig. 24.1). Spigelian hernias are difficult to diagnose since the hernia sac may lie between muscle layers, and therefore there may be no discernable mass on physical exam (Fig. 24.2). A **rectus diastasis** is not truly a hernia; it describes an acquired thinning and widening of the linea alba, which allows the abdominal contents to protrude outward. Since there is no fascial defect, on physical exam the bulge has no discernable edges.

An **incisional hernia** is a hernia through a prior surgical site that occurs when the fascia does not heal properly (Fig. 24.3a). Incisional hernias may be the result of a technical failure, such as poor closure technique and excessive tension. However, even properly closed wounds can result in a

U. Sarpel, *Surgery: An Introductory Guide*,
DOI 10.1007/978-1-4939-0903-2_24,
© Springer Science+Business Media New York 2014

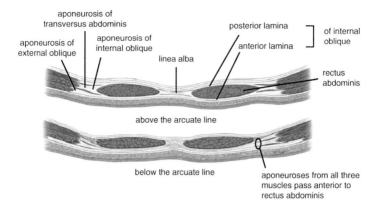

FIG. 24.1 Cross sectional diagram of the fascial layers of the anterior abdominal wall above and below the arcuate line [Reprinted from Prendergast PM. Anatomy of the Anterior Abdominal Wall. In: Shiffman MA, Di Giuseppe A (eds). Cosmetic Surgery: Art and Techniques. Heidelberg, Germany: Springer Verlag; 2013: 57–68. With permission from Springer Verlag]

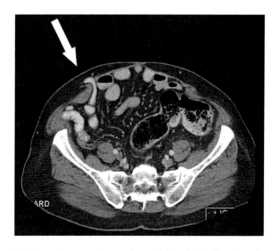

FIG. 24.2 CT scan image of a patient with a Spigelian hernia containing small bowel, as evidenced by the presence of oral contrast

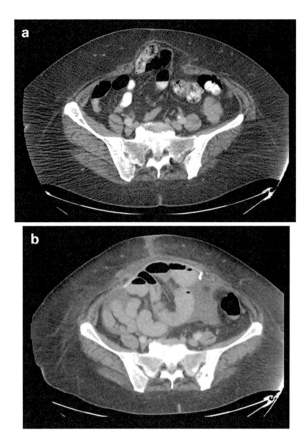

FIG. 24.3 CT scan image of a patient with (**a**) an incisional hernia at the lower pole of a prior midline incision, and (**b**) appearance after ventral hernia repair with mesh

postoperative hernia if the fascia is compromised by a wound infection. Since, by definition, incisional hernias involve prior surgery, their repair is often complicated by the presence of intra-abdominal adhesions. The repair of an incisional hernia may require an extensive lysis of adhesions before the hernia repair can begin.

The main reason to repair a hernia is to prevent the chance of incarceration or strangulation. Another important reason to perform herniorrhaphy is to prevent progression of the hernia. The constant pressure exerted by the intra-abdominal organs leads to gradual enlargement of the hernia defect. In extreme cases, the entire bowel and other intra-abdominal organs can herniate out the fascial defect. The abdominal cavity gradually contracts, and eventually can no longer contain all the abdominal contents—a phenomenon known as **loss of domain**. Sudden replacement of the viscera back into the abdomen at the time of hernia repair can lead to excessive tension and compartment syndrome. Therefore, giant hernias present a surgical challenge that often requires complex repair including abdominal relaxing incisions and large pieces of mesh.

A clinically important type of hernia, known as a **Richter's hernia**, occurs when only a small portion of the bowel wall is incarcerated within a fascial defect. Since the lumen of the bowel remains open, a patient with a Richter's hernia will not develop bowel obstruction. However, the portion of bowel wall that is trapped within the hernia can go on to become ischemic and necrotic, leading to perforation and abdominal sepsis. A delay in diagnosis often occurs in these cases since patients do not present with the typical obstructive symptoms or an obvious hernia mass on exam. Thus, a high level of suspicion is required to diagnose a Richter's hernia before strangulation occurs.

Surgical Technique

When performing an open repair of a ventral hernia, a skin incision is made and the subcutaneous fat is divided until the hernia sac is reached. The sac is freed from its attachments and followed down to the fascia, which is exposed circumferentially. The hernia sac is dissected free from the fascial edges and is reduced back into the abdomen. In elective cases, the hernia sac may be left intact, or can be opened to examine the hernia contents. In cases of acute incarceration, the sac must be opened to ensure that the contents are viable. Once the hernia has been reduced, the size of the fascial defect can be assessed. Primary repair—or direct closure of the fascial defect without mesh—should be reserved for cases in which the fascial defect is smaller than 2 cm in diameter. In this situation, the fascia is re-approximated and sutured together, thereby closing the defect.

Most ventral hernias require the use of synthetic mesh because there is either a sizable fascial defect, or because the fascia is significantly attenuated. Mesh can be used in different ways, being placed either above, below, or within the rectus sheath, per surgeon preference. The key to ventral hernia repair is to find quality fascia to which the mesh can be anchored. Successful repair may require the use of a large piece of mesh that spans much of the anterior abdominal wall to allow ample overlap with the fascia (Fig. 24.3b). In hernias where significant subcutaneous dissection was performed, a drain may be placed above the fascial closure to eliminate dead space and prevent the accumulation of fluid.

Ventral hernias are well suited to laparoscopic repair since the entire abdominal wall can be visualized and broadly covered with mesh while minimizing the size of the incision. For laparoscopic herniorrhaphy, ports are placed out laterally, away from the fascial defect. Any bowel or omentum trapped within the hernia is reduced and a lysis of adhesions is performed as needed. The hernia sac is excised to prevent seroma formation, which can occur due to the normal production of fluid from the peritoneal cells that line the hernia sac. A large piece of mesh is rolled up and inserted into the abdominal cavity via one of the trocars. The mesh is centered over the defect and secured into place. The mesh can be anchored with a laparoscopic tacking device or with sutures (Fig. 24.4).

Complications

As in any situation where a foreign body is implanted, a **mesh infection** can occur following hernia repair. Once mesh has been contaminated by bacteria, it cannot be re-sterilized even

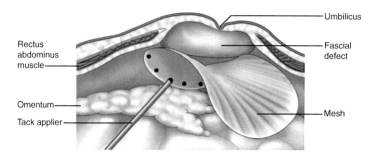

FIG. 24.4 Surgical technique for laparoscopic incisional hernia repair: rectus abdominus muscle, fascial defect, umbilicus, and mesh

with intravenous antibiotics. Therefore a mesh infection almost always requires removal of the mesh in order for the infection to resolve. Infection of the mesh is uncommon in general, but is even more rare in laparoscopic surgery as compared to open repair. Since open surgery involves greater dissection of the subcutaneous fat, dead space created is in the process and predisposes the site to wound infections. Although hernia repair is technically a clean case, pre-incision antibiotics are generally given to help in reducing the chance of infection.

The most feared complication of ventral hernia repair is an unrecognized injury to the bowel. An **inadvertent enterotomy** classically occurs during incisional hernia repair where extensive lysis of adhesions is required. Bowel can be injured by excessive traction or by thermal damage. Unfortunately, the injury is usually not appreciated at the time of surgery, and manifests days later with abdominal pain, fever, and peritonitis due to leakage of enteric contents into the abdomen. This is a devastating complication that requires immediate re-exploration, washout, explantation of the mesh, bowel resection, and possible diverting stoma, depending on the location of the injury.

As with any hernia repair, **recurrence** of the hernia is a possibility, and is always disappointing for both the patient and surgeon alike. The liberal use of mesh has significantly reduced the risk of recurrence, and in the era of mesh the most common reason for recurrence is due to improper anchoring of the mesh, insufficient overlap with healthy fascia, or excessive tension on the repair.

Classic Case

A 65-year-old woman undergoes an elective sigmoidectomy for recurrent diverticulitis, after which she develops a wound infection. Several of the skin staples are removed and copious purulent material is evacuated. The wound infection resolves, she has an otherwise uneventful recovery, and is discharged home. Over the next few weeks the wound granulates in and heals closed.

Several months later at a follow-up appointment, the surgeon notices a fascial defect and hernia at the incision site. The patient is scheduled for a laparoscopic incisional hernia repair. At surgery, adhesions from her previous operation are noted. An extensive lysis of adhesions is performed, after which the bowel is carefully examined to ensure no enterotomies have occurred. A portion of omentum which is adherent to the hernia sac is reduced. A large piece of synthetic mesh is inserted into the abdominal cavity and tacked into place along the entire perimeter.

OR Questions

1. Which is more dangerous, a hernia with a small or a large fascial defect?
   A large defect tends to allow bowel to reduce easily, whereas a small defect is more likely to cause incarceration and strangulation.
2. What imaging test should be performed to confirm the diagnosis of an incarcerated hernia in a patient who presents with an incisional mass and bowel obstruction?
   None, the patient should be taken to the operating room for immediate operative repair. A CT scan is both unnecessary

and dangerous since the time delay may lead to ischemia of the hernia contents.

3. A patient with an incisional hernia is scheduled for elective laparoscopic repair with mesh. The patient also has a history of cholecystitis and requests that cholecystectomy be performed at the same operation. What should the surgeon advise?

   Although unlikely, the possibility of mesh contamination by bacteria in the biliary tract is concerning. The surgeon should consider a laparoscopic cholecystectomy, followed by laparoscopic herniorrhaphy at a separate date.

4. During a laparoscopic hernia repair an inadvertent enterotomy is made during the lysis of adhesions and is recognized immediately. After repairing the enterotomy, how should the surgeon proceed?

   Due to the increased risk of mesh infection, a synthetic mesh should not be used in any case where there has been contamination by enteric contents. In this situation, the surgeon can perform a primary repair if feasible, or can abort the procedure and reschedule the repair for another time. The use of biologic mesh, which is composed of organic tissue, can also be considered, although these types of mesh are not as durable as synthetic meshes.

5. What distinguishes a strangulated hernia from an incarcerated one?

   The key distinction is that the contents of an incarcerated are trapped, but are not ischemic. The presence of systemic signs such as fever, tachycardia, or leukocytosis, along with the finding of erythema, tenderness, or crepitus at the site are all indicative of strangulation. No attempt at reduction should be made if these signs are present.

6. The parents of a 6-month-old bring their baby in for evaluation of an umbilical hernia. What is the recommended treatment?

   Umbilical hernias are common in children and usually close spontaneously by 2 years of age. No repair is necessary unless there are signs of incarceration.

Ventral Hernia Repair

Introduction

- Umbilical hernia: congenital defect at umbilicus
- Epigastric hernia: upper midline defect
- Incisional hernia: defect at surgical site
- Spigelian hernia: defect at edge of rectus muscle, below arcuate line where posterior sheath is absent
- Rectus diastasis: acquired thinning and widening of the linea alba, no actual fascial defect
- Loss of domain: contraction of the abdominal cavity which occurs when a massive hernia contains most of the abdominal contents
- Richter's hernia: only a portion of the bowel wall is incarcerated in the fascial defect; the bowel lumen remains patent and therefore patients do not present w/ bowel obstruction

Technique: Open repair

- Skin incision and identification of hernia sac
- Fascial edges are identified and dissected
- In cases of incarceration, the hernia sac must be opened to ensure that the contents are viable
- Small defects can be closed primarily, but most cases require the use of synthetic mesh
- Mesh can be placed either above, below, or within the rectus sheath
- Drain placement may be required if extensive dissection of subcutaneous space was performed

Technique: Laparoscopic repair
- Pneumoperitoneum is established and ports are placed far laterally
- Lysis of adhesions, as needed
- Hernia contents are reduced
- The hernia sac is excised
- A large piece of mesh is introduced
- The mesh is centered around the fascial defect
- Mesh is secured into place with tacks or sutures

Peri-op orders
- Pre-incision antibiotics are typically given if mesh is being used
- General anesthesia
- No heavy lifting for 4-6 weeks

Complications
- Mesh infection
- Inadvertent enterotomy
- Recurrence

Suggested Reading

Katkhouda N. Advanced laparoscopic surgery: techniques and tips. 2nd ed. Berlin: Springer; 2010. p. 69–180 [Chapter 11, Incisional and Ventral Hernia Repair Including Component Separation].

25
Surgical Airway

Introduction

The creation of a surgical airway by directly accessing the trachea is most often indicated in one of two situations, (1) chronically ventilator-dependent patients who require a durable airway and (2) patients with an acute loss of airway patency who require an emergency airway.

The need for a **tracheostomy** is commonly encountered in the intensive care unit when a critically ill patient is too unstable or too weak to be weaned from a ventilator. Long-term use of an oral **endotracheal tube** is associated with damage to the larynx; therefore, patients who are estimated to require mechanical ventilation for more than 2 weeks should undergo early tracheostomy.

Although sometimes family members may be resistant to the idea of a tracheostomy, this procedure actually provides several benefits to the patient. A tracheostomy facilitates weaning from the ventilator, since—by shortening the amount of tubing required in the circuit—the work of breathing is significantly decreased. Also, by eliminating the tubing in the mouth, a tracheostomy allows for better oral hygiene and is more comfortable for the patient, thus reducing sedation requirements. A tracheostomy allows for more effective control of airway secretions, thereby improving oxygenation. Finally, as the patient's status improves, a tracheostomy can be fitted with a speaking valve, which allows

U. Sarpel, *Surgery: An Introductory Guide*,   279
DOI 10.1007/978-1-4939-0903-2_25,
© Springer Science+Business Media New York 2014

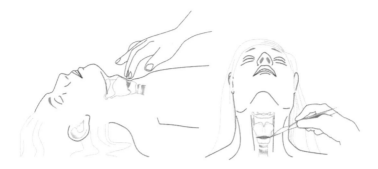

F<small>IG</small>. 25.1 Depiction of an emergency cricothyroidotomy; note that the incision is through the cricothyroid membrane [Reprinted from Lennquist S. Incidents Caused by Physical Trauma. In: Lennquist S (ed). Medical Response to Major Incidents and Disasters: A Practical Guide for All Medical Staff. Heidelberg, Germany: Springer Verlag; 2012: 111-196. With permission from Springer Verlag]

the patient to speak, without compromising the presence of a secure airway.

While a tracheostomy is the most secure airway, it is difficult to perform in emergency situations. An urgent airway may be required in any situation where patency of the airway is compromised, such as in anaphylaxis, aspiration of a foreign body, failed attempts at orotracheal intubation, or massive facial trauma. In the setting of extensive injury to the face and mouth, even if the airway itself is patent, the presence of blood and debris can hinder the visualization required for oral intubation. In these situations, a **cricothyroidotomy** allows rapid bypass of the oropharynx, thus restoring normal air supply (Fig. 25.1). A cricothyroidotomy is made higher up in the neck than a tracheostomy, through the cricothyroid membrane. This allows for rapid access to the airway, with minimal surgical equipment, and without the need to hyperextend the neck. While cricothyroidotomy has the benefit of being easier to perform, its long-term use is associated with **subglottic stenosis**, a type of airway stricture. Therefore, patients who require intubation for longer than approximately 3 days should undergo conversion to a formal tracheostomy, which is a more durable airway.

Surgical Technique

The procedure for a tracheostomy begins by positioning the patient with hyperextension of the neck to allow for access to the lower tracheal rings. Either a vertical or transverse skin incision can be used. The platysma is divided, and the underlying strap muscles are spread apart at the midline. The thyroid isthmus is identified and gently retracted upward or divided as needed to visualize the second or third tracheal ring (Fig. 25.2). An opening is made in the trachea by incising the center of a tracheal ring and spreading the trachea open. The patient's oral endotracheal tube is slowly backed out and the tracheostomy tube is inserted in through the trachea. The balloon is inflated, the tracheostomy is connected to the ventilator, the presence of end-tidal CO_2 is confirmed, and the

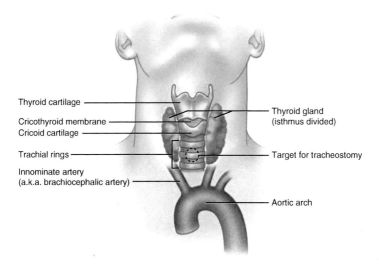

FIG. 25.2 Surgical anatomy for creation of a tracheostomy: sternohyoid muscle, omohyoid muscle, thyroid cartilage, cricoid cartilage, cricothyroid membrane, tracheal rings, thyroid isthmus, and innominate artery

tracheostomy is secured in place. The skin and subcutaneous tissues can be loosely approximated or left open to heal by granulation.

A **percutaneous tracheostomy** placement can be performed in patients with favorable neck anatomy. For this procedure, a needle is passed through the skin in the neck, and aspiration of air into the syringe confirms the location of the trachea. Once access is obtained, a wire is guided through the needle, and the tract is dilated up to match the size of a tracheostomy tube. Bronchoscopic guidance can also be used to facilitate the procedure.

In situations where a patient is actively hypoxic and requires an urgent airway, the positioning and surgical technique used for a tracheostomy would be too time consuming and a cricothryroidotomy should be performed instead. The surgeon must rely on external landmarks and a sound knowledge of neck anatomy to rapidly establish an airway. A vertical skin incision is made and the prominent thyroid cartilage is palpated. The soft cricothyroid membrane which lies between the thyroid and cricoid cartilages is identified and incised. A tracheostomy tube is inserted through the opening and secured in place.

Complications

The most obvious risk of a tracheostomy or cricothyroidotomy is subsequent loss of the airway, resulting in patient hypoxia. If a tracheostomy tube becomes dislodged early in the postoperative period, the tract may not yet be well-formed enough to allow simple reinsertion of the tube into the trachea. In these situations, standard orotracheal intubation should be performed.

Hemorrhage during a tracheostomy procedure can occur by inadvertent injury to the thyroid gland or any of the numerous nearby vessels. Dramatic, life-threatening bleeding can occur later in the postoperative period as a result of fistula formation between the trachea and the innominate artery, called a **tracheo-innominate fistula**.

Another potential complication of tracheostomy is injury to the esophagus. While the anterior aspect of the trachea contains stiff cartilaginous rings, it is important to remember that the posterior aspect of the trachea is soft, and that the esophagus lies just behind. Inadvertent injury to the esophagus can occur if the surgeon's incision into the trachea goes deep, or if the tracheostomy tube is inserted into position too roughly.

A rare but alarming risk of upper airway surgery is that of an **operating room fire**, caused by the use of electrocautery in the presence of highly oxygenated air and flammable skin prep solution. To avoid this complication, is it important to allow all prep solutions to dry, to decrease the oxygen content of the ventilated gas, and only use electrocautery as needed.

Classic Case

A 38-year-old male is brought into the emergency room following a self-inflicted gunshot wound to the face during a suicide attempt. Upon examination, the patient has massive trauma to the oropharynx. The paramedics were unable to obtain a good seal with the bag-valve mask and an oral intubation attempt was unsuccessful due to the presence of active bleeding obscuring the field. Upon arrival the patient is hypoxic and unresponsive.

The surgeon rapidly makes an incision in the neck and identifies the thyroid cartilage and the cricothyroid membrane inferior to it. A cricothyroidotomy is performed and a tracheostomy tube is inserted into the airway. The bag-valve device is connected to the tube, and the patient is ventilated with return of normal oxygen saturation levels.

Once stabilized, the patient is taken to the operating room for assessment of his injuries. It is determined that multiple complex operations will be needed to treat his facial injuries and restore function. A conversion to a formal tracheostomy is performed. Once his reconstructive surgeries are complete, the patient's tracheostomy tube is decannulated.

OR Questions

1. What criteria are used to determine if a ventilated patient can be extubated?

   No guidelines can perfectly predict whether a patient will tolerate extubation. However in general, if a patient can initiate spontaneous breaths, achieve adequate tidal volumes, and tolerate the work of breathing, it is likely that extubation will be successful.

2. A morbidly obese patient requires a tracheostomy. Which technique should be employed?

   An open tracheostomy. The percutaneous approach should be reserved for patients in whom anatomic landmarks of the neck can be easily palpated.

3. One week following tracheostomy, massive bright red bleeding develops in and around the tracheostomy tube. What is the diagnosis?

   Erosion of the tracheostomy tube into the innominate artery, known as a trachea-innominate fistula. This event is often preceded by a minor sentinel bleed that may have gone unnoticed.

4. How should this complication be managed?

   The balloon of the tracheostomy tube should be hyperinflated in an attempt to tamponade the site of bleeding. If this is unsuccessful, removal of the tracheostomy tube and digital compression against the sternum from within the tracheostomy stoma should be attempted. Definitive repair is performed in the operating room, where a sternotomy is performed to access the innominate artery.

5. A chronically ventilator-dependent patient is being moved when the tracheostomy tube becomes dislodged. What options are available to ventilate the patient?

   If the tracheostomy tract is well established, reintubation of the stoma may be successful. If not, an oral endotracheal intubation should be attempted. Ventilation using bag-valve mask should be performed to maintain oxygenation until the airway is secure.

6. Is pulmonary toilet better with an endotracheal or tracheostomy tube?
   A tracheostomy facilitates more thorough suctioning of the airway since it bypasses the oropharynx and allows access to the lower trachea and bronchi.

Surgical Airway

Indications
- Prolonged ventilator dependence
- Bypass of upper airway due to obstruction (e.g. tumor, goiter, bilateral vocal cord paralysis)
- Maxofacial trauma

Timing
- Tracheostomy should be performed early if prolonged ventilator support (>14 days) is anticipated
- Benefits include decreased work of breathing, better control of secretions, allowing for patient speech

Technique: Cricothyroidotomy
- Emergency airway
- Rapid vertical neck incision
- Incision into cricothyroid membrane
- Insertion of endotracheal tube
- Should convert to tracheostomy as soon as feasible: the high position in the neck creates risk for subglottic stenosis of trachea

Technique: Surgical tracheostomy
- Horizontal or vertical incision
- Division of platysma
- Strap muscles are spread apart
- 2nd or 3rd tracheal ring is identified
- Segment of tracheal ring is excised
- Oral endotracheal tube is withdrawn and tracheostomy tube is inserted
- Balloon inflated
- Position is confirmed with CO_2 detection

Peri-op orders:
- Hyperextend neck
- Decrease ventilator O_2 concentration to reduce the risk of a fire in the operating room
- Secure tube well prior to moving patient, since dislodgement will result in loss of airway

Complications
- Early hemorrhage: due to injury to anterior jugular vein, thyroid isthmus, or thyroid ima artery
- Late hemorrhage: due to of tracheostomy tube into erosion into innominate artery, often heralded by a sentinel bleed
- Tube dislodgement
- Esophageal injury

Suggested Reading

Yu KCY. Airway management & tracheotomy. In: Lalwani AK, editor. CURRENT diagnosis & treatment in otolaryngology—head & neck surgery. 3rd ed. New York: McGraw-Hill Professional Publishing; 2012.

26
Trauma Laparotomy

Introduction

The abdominal organs, given their central location and lack of bony protection, are vulnerable to traumatic injury. The type of trauma can predict the pattern of injuries that are likely to have occurred. In **blunt abdominal trauma**—such as a fall from height, motor vehicle collision, or physical assault—the liver and the spleen are the most commonly damaged organs. The force of impact can cause these solid organs to fracture, leading to **intra-abdominal hemorrhage**. When examining a victim of blunt trauma, sites of ecchymosis on the abdominal wall can demonstrate points of impact and identify likely underlying organ injury. Bedside ultrasound, called the **Focused Assessment with Sonography for Trauma** (**FAST**) exam, can be used to assess for intra-abdominal bleeding. Visualization of a black hypoechoic stripe along the paracolic gutters or pelvic cul-de-sac indicates the presence of free fluid in the abdominal cavity.

Even in the presence of intra-abdominal bleeding, advances in supportive care have allowed the majority of blunt trauma patients to be spared operative exploration. In clinically stable patients, CT imaging is useful in identifying the extent of **splenic laceration** or **liver laceration** (Fig. 26.1). Minor intra-abdominal bleeding is typically self-limited, but if extravasation of intravenous contrast is seen, this indicates active bleeding that is unlikely to resolve. Interventional radiology techniques can be used to selectively embolize

U. Sarpel, *Surgery: An Introductory Guide*,
DOI 10.1007/978-1-4939-0903-2_26,
© Springer Science+Business Media New York 2014

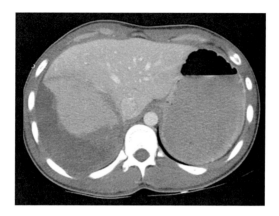

FIG. 26.1 CT scan of a patient who was involved in a motor vehicle accident, the images demonstrate a large liver laceration with accompanying hemoperitoneum. The patient remained hemodynamically stable and operative intervention was not required

these bleeding vessels. Patients who remain hemodynamically unstable despite these efforts, or who continue to require blood products for resuscitation should be taken to the operating room for definitive control of bleeding sites.

In contrast to blunt trauma, **penetrating abdominal trauma** is more likely to result in injuries that require surgical intervention. With stabbing injuries, damage will occur to whichever organs lie in the path of the weapon, often including the bowel and major blood vessels. The finding of frank peritonitis on examination implies bowel injury with the spillage of enteric contents and mandates operative exploration. If no peritonitis is present, wound sites can be explored at bedside to determine if the peritoneal cavity has been violated. With stabbings, it is important to keep in mind that the size of the skin wound does not correlate with the depth of penetration; a small skin defect may be the only indication of a deep wound with severe internal injury. CT imaging is not sensitive for identifying bowel injury. Therefore, any patient with a stab wound penetrating the peritoneum must have bowel injury ruled out with either a **peritoneal lavage** or operative exploration (Fig. 26.2).

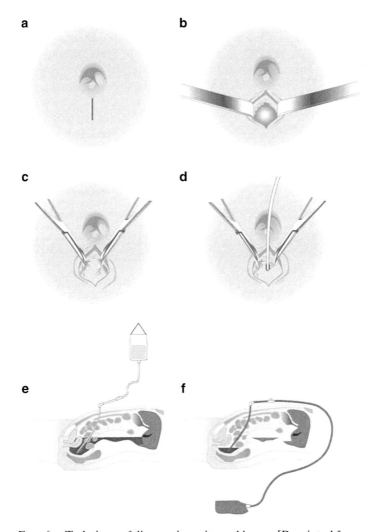

FIG. 26.2 Technique of diagnostic peritoneal lavage [Reprinted from Lennquist S. Incidents Caused by Physical Trauma. In: Lennquist S (ed). Medical Response to Major Incidents and Disasters: A Practical Guide for All Medical Staff. Heidelberg, Germany: Springer Verlag; 2012: 111-196. With permission from Springer Verlag]

Gunshot wounds present the potential for complex thermal and mechanical damage. The heat produced by a bullet causes direct thermal injury to the surrounding structures. In addition, the tumbling of the bullet can cause more extensive damage than anticipated. Complex, multi-organ injury is virtually guaranteed with a gunshot wound to the abdomen, and as such all patients should be taken directly for operative exploration.

Surgical Technique

A generous midline incision is employed for a trauma laparotomy since this provides rapid access to the abdomen with good exposure to all potentially injured organs. Once the abdominal cavity is opened, an initial survey is quickly performed. If blood is present, multiple laparotomy pads are used to pack all four quadrants for control of hemorrhage. Bowel injuries causing gross spillage of enteric contents are provisionally closed to limit contamination. After initial damage control is obtained, a careful examination of the abdomen is conducted; packing is sequentially removed, and each quadrant is systematically inspected for injury.

Major vascular injuries take priority and are addressed by obtaining inflow and outflow control, and performing repair as appropriate. Stable retroperitoneal or pelvic hematomas are typically left undisturbed, since opening the retroperitoneum can decompress the space and disrupt hemostasis. Embolization of the pelvic arteries can be performed in interventional radiology to assist with control of the pelvic hematomas seen with extensive pelvic fractures.

The liver has a unique ability to achieve hemostasis, therefore bleeding from liver lacerations is usually self-limited or can be controlled with simple compression. In more serious injuries, a **Pringle maneuver** can be performed to control the blood inflow to the liver. By encircling the porta hepatis and applying manual pressure, the surgeon can occlude the portal vein and hepatic artery, and allow visualization of injuries (Fig. 26.3).

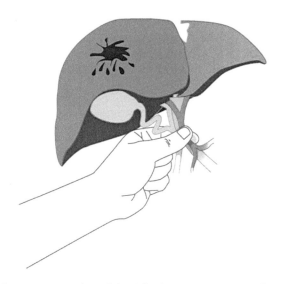

FIG. 26.3 Demonstration of the Pringle maneuver: manual occlusion of the portal vein, hepatic artery, and common bile duct to obtain inflow control to the liver. [Reprinted from Lennquist S. Incidents Caused by Physical Trauma. In: Lennquist S (ed). Medical Response to Major Incidents and Disasters: A Practical Guide for All Medical Staff. Heidelberg, Germany: Springer Verlag; 2012: 111-196. With permission from Springer Verlag]

Active arterial bleeding may require ligation of the hepatic artery to the bleeding lobe. Emergent liver resection is only rarely needed, but may be indicated for ongoing hemorrhage or a significant bile leak.

Splenic lacerations can be addressed either by performing a **splenectomy** or attempting splenic repair. **Splenorrhaphy** — or repair of an injured spleen — can be considered in stable patients, and particularly in children, for whom splenic function remains more important. Splenectomy is the fastest and most definitive way to achieve hemostasis, and should be performed without hesitation in the setting of significant hemorrhage or failed **splenic embolization**.

In order to identify any bowel injuries, a thorough examination of the entire length of the intra-abdominal GI tract must be conducted. Small punctures and lacerations may be debrided and closed primarily. However, in the setting of crush injuries or gunshot wounds, it is important to remember that the zone of devitalized tissue extends past the visible damage. In these cases, a bowel resection and anastomosis to healthy tissue should be performed. Diversion with either an ileostomy or colostomy should be performed as needed.

Complications

Operations for complex trauma can lead to severe physiologic derangements including the triad of **hypothermia, acidosis, and coagulopathy**. Long operative times and exposed surfaces lead to the rapid loss of body heat. Concomitant blood transfusions and large-volume fluid resuscitation cause acidosis and dilution of clotting factors—further exacerbating the coagulopathy. If acidosis and coagulopathy occur, it is best to halt the operation, temporarily close the abdomen, and transfer the patient to the intensive care unit. Once the hypothermia, acidosis, and coagulopathy have been reversed, the patient can be brought back to the operating room for definitive repair of injuries and abdominal closure.

The most serious complication of a trauma laparotomy is an incomplete assessment of the abdomen resulting in a **missed injury**. Despite the time pressure and air of chaos that can sometimes accompany severe traumas, it is imperative that the surgeon identifies all sites of damage. The most common missed injury is a small enterotomy. This type of injury can be easily missed by blood or enteric contents obscuring visualization. The consequences of a missed enterotomy are potentially fatal, and underscore the need to "run the bowel" meticulously—and preferably twice—prior to closure.

Diffuse bowel edema can develop during a trauma laparotomy due to the massive fluid resuscitation that trauma

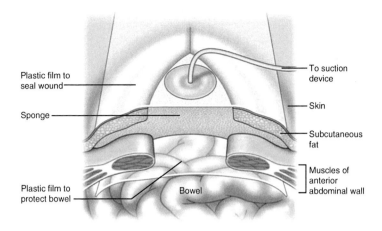

Plastic film to
seal wound

To suction
device

Sponge

Skin

Subcutaneous
fat

Muscles of
anterior
abdominal wall

Plastic film to
protect bowel

Bowel

FIG. 26.4 Technique for use of a negative pressure dressing for an open abdomen following trauma laparotomy: bowel is protected with a plastic film, a sponge is applied to fill the wound, the wound is sealed with a second layer of plastic, tubing is placed over a hole in the plastic and connected to a suction device. The negative pressure created by the suction evacuates blood and fluid and also aids in wound contraction

patients often receive. If excessive tension is used to force the fascia closed, an abdominal **compartment syndrome** can result. The elevated intra-abdominal pressure on the inferior vena cava leads to diminished venous return and decreased cardiac output. The high pressure and hypoperfusion also cause acute renal injury with oliguria and rising creatinine. In addition, the edematous bowel may displace the diaphragms superiorly, interfering with normal pulmonary function. Peak airway pressures can be used for monitoring of excessive tension as the fascia is being closed.

   If bowel edema precludes closure of the fascia, the abdomen should be left open with a temporary dressing to cover the abdominal contents (Fig. 26.4). In most cases, as the patient recovers and mobilizes excess fluid, the bowel edema will resolve and allow formal closure of the abdomen within a few days. Dressing changes on an **open abdomen** must be managed carefully since the intestines are exposed and vulnerable to damage.

Classic Case

A 23-year-old male is brought into the trauma bay following an assault. Upon arrival the patient is awake and alert. He reports being stabbed several times with a knife and is complaining of diffuse abdominal pain. The patient is connected to monitors and large-bore peripheral intravenous access is established in both arms. He is tachycardic to 130 bpm, but is normotensive. One liter of isotonic fluid is initiated, and his heart rate drops to 110 bpm. On examination, breath sounds are noted to be equal bilaterally and a bedside chest X-ray confirms the absence of a pneumothorax. The patient's abdomen is non-distended, but guarding and tenderness are present. Three stab wounds are identified: one in the right midclavicular line just above the costal margin, one in the epigastrium, and one in the periumbilical region. Omentum is seen protruding from the most inferior wound.

Once the primary survey is complete, the patient is taken to the operating room for exploration. Upon entering the abdomen, a large amount of blood is encountered. The blood is suctioned out and all four quadrants are quickly packed with laparotomy pads. On closer examination, the bleeding is localized to a liver laceration. A Pringle maneuver is performed and hemostasis is achieved with suture ligation and electrocautery. Exploration of the remainder of the abdomen reveals a puncture of the anterior wall of the stomach, and a laceration of the small bowel. The stomach injury is debrided and repaired primarily; the small bowel is handled with a resection and anastomosis. After reexamination of the liver to confirm hemostasis, the abdomen is irrigated and closed. The patient has an uneventful postoperative recovery and is ultimately discharged home.

OR Questions

1. What percentage of total blood volume is lost before a patient will exhibit hypotension?
   Hypotension is a sign of advanced hemorrhage and does not manifest until over 30 % of the circulating blood volume has been lost. In an adult this represents blood loss of over 1 L.

2. What type of intravenous fluid should be used for resuscitation of a trauma victim?
   An isotonic fluid should be employed initially; O-negative blood should be used in cases of massive hemorrhage or ongoing blood loss.

3. What is a "transient responder"?
   A patient whose tachycardia initially responds to volume resuscitation, but then deteriorates again, this hemodynamic pattern implies ongoing hemorrhage.

4. Which is the preferred access to resuscitate a patient in hemorrhagic shock, a large-bore peripheral IV, or a triple lumen central line?
   A large-bore peripheral line has a wider diameter and offers less resistance than a central line, and therefore will allow more rapid infusion of fluids and blood products, as demonstrated by Poiseuille's law.

5. A patient who is involved in a motor vehicle accident sustains complex pelvic fractures and is tachycardic and hypotensive upon arrival to the hospital. Abdominal exam is benign and FAST does not reveal intra-abdominal fluid. What it the appropriate treatment?
   Rapid administration of intravenous fluids and blood, a pelvic compression device, and emergent embolization of pelvic vessels in interventional radiology.

6. A clinically stable patient with a single stab wound to the left flank should undergo what kind of imaging?
   Injury to retroperitoneal structures can be assessed with a CT of the abdomen/pelvis. Intravenous contrast allows evaluation of the kidney and GU tract. The addition of rectal contrast facilitates visualization of injury to the retroperitoneal portion of the descending colon.

7. A multi-trauma patient undergoes massive transfusions
   during surgery; ultimately hemostasis is achieved and the
   abdomen is closed. Postoperatively in the SICU the patient
   is hypotensive, oliguric with high peak airway pressures.
   Lab tests demonstrate rising creatinine and lactate levels.
   What is the diagnosis and treatment?
   *The suspicion of abdominal compartment syndrome can be
   confirmed by measuring the intra-abdominal pressure via
   a transducer in the bladder. If the pressures exceed 25
   mmHg, the patient should be emergently taken back to the
   operating room and the abdomen reopened.*

Trauma Laparotomy

Blunt abdominal trauma

- Assault, motor vehicle collision, fall from height, crush injury
- The majority of patients can be managed non-operatively
- CT imaging useful in assessing extent of injuries
- Most common injury is solid-organ fracture, such as a splenic or liver laceration
- Embolization can be used to control bleeding, from the spleen or pelvic vessels

Penetrating abdominal trauma

- Stabbing, gunshot, shrapnel injury
- More often requires operative management
- Size of skin wound does not correlate with depth of penetration or extent of intra-abdominal injury
- CT imaging less useful, since it is insensitive for detection of bowel injuries

Technique

- Vertical midline incision
- Four-quadrant packing
- Obtain hemostasis
- "Run the bowel"
- Repair of injuries as required
- Ileostomy/colostomy if indicated
- Abdominal closure if no significant bowel edema

Peri-op orders

- Careful monitoring of urine output and creatinine if compartment syndrome is of concern
- Advance diet as appropriate for procedure
- Vaccinations given two weeks post-op if splenectomy was performed

Complications

- Hypothermia, acidosis, and coagulopathy
- Missed injury
- Abdominal compartment syndrome
- Open abdomen

Suggested Reading

Hirshberg A. Trauma laparotomy: principles and techniques. In: Mattox KL, Moore EE, Feliciano DV, editors. Trauma. 7th ed. New York: McGraw-Hill Professional Publishing; 2013.

27
Central Venous Access

Introduction

The smaller peripheral veins in the extremities drain into the **subclavian vein**, **internal jugular vein**, and **femoral vein**, and these vessels constitute the central venous system (Fig. 27.1). The ability to create secure access to the central venous system greatly facilitates the care of many patients. One of the benefits of central venous catheterization is the ability to rapidly dilute therapeutic substances into the blood stream that would be too noxious to deliver through smaller, peripheral veins. **Total parenteral nutrition**, **chemotherapy**, and **vasopressors** are all examples of therapies that require delivery via a large central vein.

Central venous catheterization is also required for therapies such as **hemodialysis, continuous venovenous hemofiltration**, and **plasmapheresis**. In these therapies, high rates of blood flow must be generated in order to circulate the patient's entire volume of blood through an external device. This process requires a large bore catheter that can only be placed in wide diameter vessels such as the central veins.

In certain patients central venous access may be indicated for close hemodynamic monitoring. Measurement of the **central venous pressure** can be obtained through an indwelling venous catheter with a pressure transducer. This reading can be used to estimate the intravascular blood volume, which can help guide resuscitation decisions. In highly select cases,

U. Sarpel, *Surgery: An Introductory Guide*,   299
DOI 10.1007/978-1-4939-0903-2_27,
© Springer Science+Business Media New York 2014

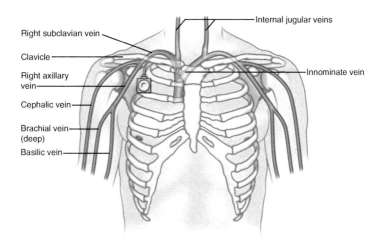

FIG. 27.1 Surgical anatomy for central venous access: internal jugular vein, innominate vein, subclavian vein, axillary vein, cephalic vein, brachial vein, and basilic vein

a **pulmonary artery catheter** may be indicated to evaluate cardiac function parameters. For this procedure, a long catheter with an inflatable balloon tip is guided into a central vein, then through the right atrium and ventricle, into the pulmonary artery. By inflating the balloon, a measurement can be obtained of the pressure in the pulmonary artery, which indirectly reflects the pressure in the left atrium. In addition, a temperature probe on the pulmonary artery catheter can be used to calculate cardiac output based on thermodilution. These measurements can help guide clinical decisions in critically ill patients.

Finally, central venous access is occasionally indicated in patients who have poor peripheral veins, usually as a result of long inpatient admissions and frequent access attempts. In such patients, central venous catheterization certainly facilitates frequent blood draws or the administration of multiple intravenous medications. However, it is important to note that central venous catheterization should be used as a last resort, and not for convenience, since it exposes the patient to significantly higher risks than peripheral venous access.

Once central venous catheterization is indicated for one of the above reasons, the next step involves choosing which vein should be used. The right and left internal jugular veins, subclavian veins, and femoral veins each have their own advantages and disadvantages that should be considered on a case-by-case basis. The internal jugular veins are generally the preferred site of access because they are associated with the lowest rates of pneumothorax. There is, however, a risk of injury to the carotid artery during this approach. In addition, external catheters on the neck can be uncomfortable for conscious patients. The subclavian veins are advantageous in certain situations: they may provide the easiest access in obese patients in whom landmarks in the neck are not visible. Subclavian line are also generally the most comfortable for the patient. On the other hand, subclavian vein puncture is technically more difficult for the novice; furthermore the vein is not accessible for direct pressure in the event of bleeding. The femoral veins provide quick, easy access with minimal risk of injury. This is particularly useful in frenzied code situations when the intubation team crowds the area around the patient's head. The femoral veins are also preferred in coagulopathic patients since the site can be compressed with direct pressure. The disadvantage of femoral venous access is that these lines may be more prone to infection. In addition, the location of femoral catheters generally prevents ambulation.

The type of venous access catheter that is selected depends on the indication and anticipated duration of use. Simple external catheters, such as **triple lumen catheters**, are the best choice for patients who require short-term central venous access during their hospital stay. In general, these lines must be changed every few days to prevent infection. External catheters are not appropriate for outpatients due to the risk of air embolism if the catheter is inadvertently dislodged.

Peripherally inserted central catheters (**PICC**) are a special type of central line. These long catheters are inserted via the basilic vein in the upper arm, but the tip of the line is

located in the superior vena cava. These types of catheters are
well suited to outpatients who require days to weeks of intravenous access, such as commonly needed for antibiotic
administration.

Tunneled catheters are central lines that are passed
through a subcutaneous tunnel before their exit site on the
skin. A felt cuff is usually present on the catheter; tissue infil-
tration of the cuff seals the tunnel site and helps prevent
bacterial migration from the skin. These semi-permanent
catheters are ideal for patients who require several weeks or
months of central venous access, such as patients undergoing
plasmaphoresis or hemodialysis.

Subcutaneous ports are completely internalized venous
access devices. The venous catheter is connected to a reservoir located in a subcutaneous pocket on the chest wall. The
skin over the port is punctured to gain access to the central
venous system. These implanted ports are the most resistant
to infection and are the best option for patients who may
require months or years of therapy, such as those receiving
systemic chemotherapy (Fig. 27.2).

Surgical Technique

The technique for central venous catheterization varies slightly
by location; the internal jugular vein is the most commonly
used site and is described in detail here. The patient is first
placed into **Trendelenburg position** to reduce the risk of air
embolism. Anatomic landmarks alone can be used to guide the
initial venous puncture, however the use of ultrasound is preferred since it is associated with significantly lower complication rates. On ultrasonography of the neck, the internal jugular
vein is visualized as a larger, compressible structure, while the
carotid artery is seen to have a smaller lumen, thicker wall, and
posterior position, relative to the vein (Fig. 27.3).

Once venous puncture is established, the syringe is
removed and a guide wire is passed down the lumen of the
hollow needle. The needle is removed, leaving only the guide

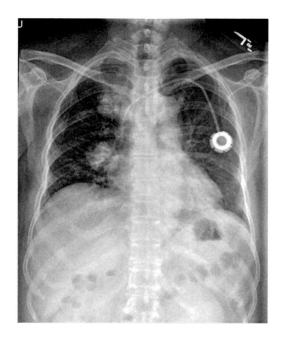

FIG. 27.2 Chest X-ray of a patient with a port placed via the left subclavian vein for the administration of systemic chemotherapy, note the presence of pulmonary metastases

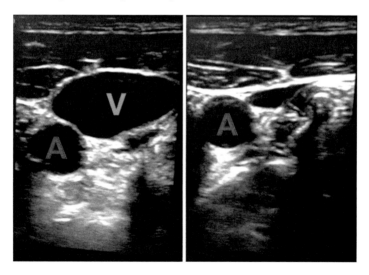

FIG. 27.3 Ultrasound of the neck demonstrating the common carotid artery (A) and internal jugular vein (V), note the collapse of the vein when gentle compression is applied

wire in the internal jugular vein. The skin at the puncture site is incised to allow entry of a dilator, which is then passed over the wire to further stretch the skin and subcutaneous tissues. Finally, the catheter is passed over the guide wire, and the wire is removed. The catheter is aspirated to ensure blood return, then flushed with saline, and sutured into position.

The same technique can be used for the placement of a subcutaneous port. After obtaining venous access as described above, a small subcutaneous pocket is created on the chest wall. The port device is positioned into the pocket and a tunnel is created from the pocket to the guide wire exit site on the neck. The port's catheter is passed through the tunnel, avoiding any sharp bends. The catheter is then trimmed to the appropriate length to ensure that its tip will rest at the junction of the superior vena cava and right atrium. Next a dilator with a break-away sheath is passed over the guide wire. Once the tract has been dilated, the dilator and wire are removed, leaving only the sheath in the vein. The port's catheter is fed through the sheath and the sheath is peeled away. Intraoperative fluoroscopy can be used to facilitate appropriate positioning of the catheter. Alternatively, direct cut down into the deltoid-pectoral groove can be used to access the cephalic vein; this approach eliminates the need for a subcutaneous tunnel.

Complications

Central venous access can be complicated by inadvertent injury to any of the surrounding structures. Puncture of the pleura can lead to a **simple pneumothorax**, while injury to the lung parenchyma itself can lead to an ongoing air leak, potentially causing a **tension pneumothorax**. Injury to the back wall of the vein may cause ongoing bleeding that can result in a **hemothorax**. A chest X-ray to assess for these complications is therefore obligatory after central line placement.

Accidental arterial puncture is another potential complication of central venous access. If the **arterial injury** is recognized immediately, the needle should be withdrawn and

direct pressure should be applied to the site for several minutes. If the arterial puncture is unrecognized, and actual can-
nulation of the artery has occurred, there is a much higher
potential for complications. In these cases, a vascular surgery
consultation should be obtained since operative repair of the
arteriotomy may be necessary. At a minimum, an ultrasound
of the artery should be performed to rule out the formation
of a pseudoaneurysm at the injury site.

Infection is a later potential complication of central
venous catheters. Meticulous sterile technique should always
be used when placing central lines; nevertheless bacteria
from the patient's skin can migrate down the catheter, leading to infection. Alternatively, bacteremia from another site
of infection can seed a venous catheter. The incidence of line
infection increases with the number of days that the catheter
has been present, therefore central lines that are no longer
necessary should be promptly removed.

The bacteremia resulting from line infections can lead to a
dramatic clinical presentation, known as **line sepsis**. Patients
may present with high fever, rigors, marked hypotension, and
leukocytosis. Patients with central venous catheters who present with sudden onset of these signs should be assumed to
have line sepsis, and therapy should not be delayed while
waiting for the results of blood cultures. The line should be
removed immediately, the tip of the catheter should be sent
for culture, and the patient should receive a dose of vancomycin. In most patients, removal of the line is sufficient treatment for line sepsis, but the need for further antibiotic
therapy should be determined on a case-by-case basis.

Finally, the removal of central venous catheters is associated
with its own potential complications. If air is allowed to enter
the venous system during removal of a central line, an **air
embolism** can occur. To prevent this potentially fatal complication, it is important to follow a strict protocol during central
line removal. Several maneuvers are performed to increase
the central venous pressure, making air entry into the vein
less likely. First, patients should be placed into the

Trendelenburg position. Next, patients should be asked to hum while the catheter is being removed. Humming acts as a Valsalva maneuver, which serves to further increase the central venous pressure and also ensures that the patient is not taking a breath in during the removal. Finally, the central line site should be covered with an occlusive dressing.

Classic Case

A 59-year-old woman who initially presented with painless jaundice is found to have a mass in the head of the pancreas. A CT scan also demonstrates the presence of numerous hepatic lesions and a liver biopsy confirms metastatic adenocarcinoma consistent with a pancreatic primary. She is referred to a medical oncologist and is found to be a good candidate for systemic chemotherapy. A surgical consultation is requested for placement of a single-lumen port. In the operating room, the patient is placed into Trendelenburg position with a rolled towel under the scapula. The right subclavian vein is first accessed with a thin finder needle, next a larger bore access needle is used for entry, and then the guide wire is passed into the lumen of the vein. The catheter is then inserted and the port positioned in its pocket.

   Immediately after the procedure, the patient reports some mild, right-sided chest pain. A postoperative chest X-ray demonstrates the presence of a small apical pneumothorax. She is administered 100 % oxygen and observed in a monitored setting. A repeat chest X-ray 6 h later shows resolution of the pneumothorax and she is discharged home. The patient returns to her medical oncologist and begins systemic chemotherapy without incident.

OR Questions

1. Why is the right internal jugular vein preferred over the left for central venous access?
   Larger diameter, more direct path to the superior vena cava, lower level of the right pleura, and absence of the thoracic duct.

2. Which bacteria are the most common cause of line sepsis?
   Coagulase negative staphylococci and staphylococcus aureus.

3. What are the anatomic landmarks for accessing the internal jugular vein?
   The internal jugular vein should be punctured at the apex of the triangle formed by the two heads of the sternocleidomastoid muscle and the clavicle.

4. What is the Seldinger technique?
   The technique of exchanging catheters over a guide wire, this method greatly facilitates safe and efficient placement of central lines.

5. What is the physiological effect of an air embolus?
   A large bubble of air in the venous system disrupts the mechanics of blood flow from the right heart into the pulmonary artery, potentially leading to hemodynamic collapse and cardiac arrest.

6. What is the treatment of a suspected air embolus?
   The patient should be placed into the Trendelenburg and left lateral decubitus position to promote accumulation of the air in the apex of the right ventricle. 100 % oxygen may promote faster reabsorption of the air embolus. An intravenous fluid bolus should be administered to maximize intravascular volume.

Central Venous Catheterization

Indications
- Chemotherapy administration
- Parenteral nutrition
- Hemodialysis
- Plasmapheresis
- Hemodynamic monitoring (e.g. pulmonary artery catheter)
- Poor peripheral venous access

Access sites
- Internal Jugular vein
- Subclavian vein
    - via cephalic vein (direct cut-down)
    - via basilic vein in arm for PICC
- Femoral vein

Types of access catheters
- External catheter: e.g. triple-lumen catheter, only for inpatient use, shortest duration (days)
- Tunneled catheter: e.g. Hickman, Permcath, Broviac, catheter exits the skin after travelling through a subcutaneous tunnel, cuff helps secure line and increases resistance to infection, medium duration (weeks-months)
- Peripherally inserted central line (PICC): long tubing enters vein in arm, but tip of catheter is in the superior vena cavavein, medium duration (weeks)
- Implantable port: e.g. Port-a-cath / Mediport, subcutaneous reservoir which is accessed by needle puncture through the overlying skin, longest life span (months-years)

Technique – External catheter
- Trendelenburg position
- Identify target vessel by surface landmarks or ultrasound (preferred)
- Seldinger technique: pass a guide wire through access needle, dilate subcutaneous tissues, then exchange catheter over guide wire
- Flush catheter and secure with sutures

Technique – Subcutaneous port
- Venous access as above
- Create subcutaneous pocket on chest wall
- Trim catheter length for proper tip position
- Tunnel catheter from subcutaneous pocket to venous access site
- Guide catheter into vein
- Secure port with sutures and close incision
- Direct cut-down onto the cephalic vein is an alternative technique

Peri-op orders
- Post-op chest x-ray to confirm position of catheter tip and rule-out pneumothorax
- Regular diet
- Ambulatory procedure

Complications
- Pneumothorax
- Hemothorax
- Arterial injury
- Line sepsis
- Air embolism

Suggested Reading

Marino PL. Establishing venous access (Chapter 6). In: Marino PL, Sutin KM, editors. The ICU book. 3rd ed. Philadelphia: Lippincott Williams & Wilkins; 2007. p. 107–28.

28

Carotid Endarterectomy

Introduction

The carotid artery is one of the main sites affected by **athero-sclerotic disease**. Plaque deposition tends to occur at sites of turbulent blood flow, in this case along the bifurcation of the common carotid artery. As the disease progresses, the enlarging plaque impinges upon the vessel lumen, causing stenosis of the carotid artery. While most patients with **carotid stenosis** will remain asymptomatic, some will experience a neurologic event due to low cerebral blood flow or embolization of plaque material. A **stroke** or **transient ischemic attack** (TIA) is the most common symptom of carotid stenosis, and typically manifests as a contralateral motor defect, sensory loss, or abnormal speech. Another sign of carotid disease is **amaurosis fugax**, an ipsilateral transient monocular blindness caused by a small embolus to the ophthalmic artery.

Patients suspected of having carotid artery disease should undergo evaluation with a **carotid duplex ultrasound**. CT or MR angiography may also be used in certain cases (Fig. 28.1). The method used to determine the degree of stenosis varies somewhat, but is typically calculated as the diameter of the most stenotic portion of the vessel compared to the diameter of the normal vessel just distal to the stenosis. A narrowing of the carotid artery lumen greater than 50 % is generally considered clinically significant.

U. Sarpel, *Surgery: An Introductory Guide*,
DOI 10.1007/978-1-4939-0903-2_28,
© Springer Science+Business Media New York 2014

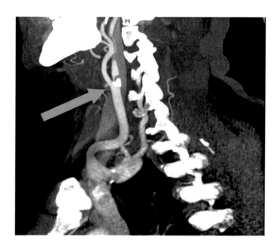

FIG. 28.1 CT angiogram image of a patient with greater than 70 % stenosis of the right carotid bulb and proximal internal carotid artery (*arrow*)

The treatment of carotid artery disease begins with lifestyle modifications such as smoking cessation, and pharmacologic therapy with aspirin and cholesterol lowering agents. Multiple randomized controlled trials have been performed to assess the efficacy of surgical **carotid endarterectomy** (CEA) in preventing future strokes over this pharmacologic therapy alone. The results of these studies indicate that the greatest benefit of endarterectomy is seen in patients who have experienced neurologic symptoms attributable to carotid disease. Patients are considered to have **symptomatic carotid stenosis** if a stroke, TIA, or amaurosis fugax has occurred within the prior 6 months. Symptomatic patients with carotid stenosis greater than 70 % have been shown to have lower future stroke rates with CEA than with medical therapy alone. In addition, CEA may have benefit in carefully selected symptomatic patients with even lower degrees of stenosis, from 50 to 70 %.

The optimal management of patients with **asymptomatic carotid stenosis** is not as clear. Earlier studies suggested that even asymptomatic patients could benefit from CEA, although the advantage was more modest than seen for symptomatic patients. However, the quality of pharmacologic therapy has improved substantially in the years since these trials were performed, thereby lowering the potential benefit margin of surgery. In addition, female patients were found to have derived less benefit than their male counterparts. As a result, recommendations for asymptomatic patients vary considerably with some surgeons recommending medical management only, and others reserving CEA for selected male patients with stenosis of greater than 60 %.

The benefit of endarterectomy assumes that the procedure itself can be performed with minimal morbidity. During clamping of the carotid artery it is imperative to ensure that the cerebral hemisphere continues to receive adequate perfusion. The vast majority of individuals will obtain sufficient cerebral blood flow from the contralateral circulation via the **Circle of Willis**. If endarterectomy is being performed under local anesthesia, the adequacy of this perfusion can be monitored in real time with ongoing assessments of the patient's mental status, speech, and extremity function. If general anesthesia is used, adequate brain perfusion can be assessed using continuous EEG monitoring. If signs of neurologic compromise are seen, an emergent carotid shunt is placed in order to restore blood flow to the cerebral hemisphere. Some surgeons prefer to use carotid shunting routinely in all patients as a method of ensuring continuous blood flow. However critics of universal shunting point out that shunts are associated with their own set of complications.

Carotid endarterectomy is considered the standard treatment for patients requiring intervention for carotid stenosis. However, symptomatic patients who have significant comorbidities and are considered to be of unacceptably high medical risk for surgery can be evaluated for **carotid artery stenting** as an alternative to CEA (Fig. 28.2). Endovascular stenting may also be preferable in patients who develop restenosis after prior surgical endarterectomy.

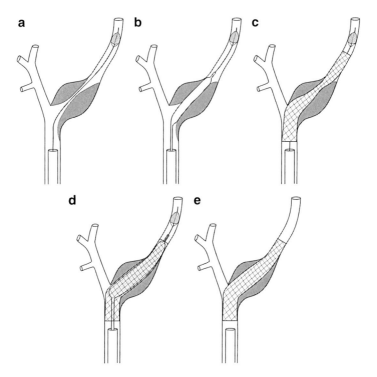

FIG. 28.2 Endovascular carotid artery stenting [Reprinted from
Goode SD, Cleveland TJ. Carotid and Vertebral Artery Intervention.
In: Cowling MG (ed). Vascular Interventional Radiology: Current
Evidence in Endovascular Surgery. Heidelberg, Germany: Springer
Verlag; 2012: 111-120. With permission from Springer Verlag]

Surgical Technique

Carotid endarterectomy begins with a neck incision along the
anterior aspect of the sternocleidomastoid muscle. The underlying platysma muscle and subcutaneous tissues are divided,
the carotid sheath is opened, and the internal jugular vein is
reflected laterally to reveal the course of the carotid artery
(Fig. 28.3). The **hypoglossal nerve** crosses just distal to the
carotid bifurcation and is carefully protected. The carotid

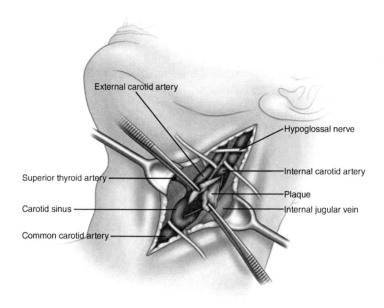

FIG. 28.3 Surgical anatomy during carotid endarterectomy: common carotid artery, carotid sinus, external carotid artery, internal carotid artery, superior thyroid artery, internal jugular vein, and hypoglossal nerve

artery is then dissected from the common trunk to its bifurcation into the internal and external arteries. Plaque formation often extends into the internal carotid, and the dissection should be carried out beyond the plaque, onto normal artery.

Vascular control is obtained by placing vessel loops around the common, internal, and external carotid artery. The patient is then given a bolus of intravenous heparin and the arteries are clamped sequentially, with the internal carotid artery being clamped first to prevent embolization. A longitudinal incision is made in the common carotid artery and extended distally into the internal carotid as needed. If routine shunting is being performed, the device is inserted into position, reestablishing flow into the internal carotid artery.

If no shunt is being used, then stump pressures of the internal carotid should be measured and the patient's neurological function is closely monitored for signs of ischemia. The atherosclerotic plaque is then carefully peeled off the wall of the carotid artery, dissecting circumferentially until free.

During closure of the arteriotomy it is recommended to patch the artery with a piece of vein or prosthetic material, in order to prevent narrowing at the closure site. Just prior to completion of the arterial closure, the clamps are briefly released to flush out any debris. After the suture line is complete, the clamps are again released, with the clamp on the internal carotid is released last, and flow is restored. Once hemostasis is ensured, the incision is closed in layers.

Complications

Cardiac complications, including **acute myocardial infarction**, are a common cause of postoperative morbidity following carotid endarterectomy. This is not surprising since all patients with carotid atherosclerosis, by definition, also have some degree of coronary artery disease. As a result, all patients being considered for CEA should undergo a thorough cardiac evaluation.

Several cranial nerves pass through the surgical field and are at risk for **nerve injury** during carotid endarterectomy, including the **marginal mandibular branch of the facial nerve**, the **hypoglossal nerve**, and the **vagus nerve** that at this level includes fibers of the **recurrent laryngeal nerve**. Fortunately, the majority of these cranial nerve injuries will resolve over several months. A strong knowledge of anatomy is imperative to preventing nerve injury.

Patients undergoing carotid endarterectomy are at risk for a postoperative **neck hematoma** owing to the extensive dissection and arterial suture line in the setting of systemic heparinization. Any patient with a neck swelling that causes tracheal deviation or who develops respiratory stridor should be immediately taken back to the operating room for hematoma evacuation and hemostasis.

Postoperative stroke may occur following endarterectomy for various reasons, including embolization of plaque material, acute arterial dissection at the endarterectomy site, or thrombosis of the anastomosis. Patients must be monitored closely after surgery and the onset of a neurologic defect should prompt immediate investigation. It is important to immediately rule out a technical problem or thrombosis at the anastomosis with urgent imaging or operative re-exploration of the site.

Hyperperfusion syndrome is a condition that occurs after endarterectomy when the cerebral hemisphere that has been accustomed to attenuated blood flow is suddenly exposed to normal perfusion pressures following correction of the carotid stenosis. This condition is more common in elderly patients with bilateral carotid stenosis. These higher perfusion pressures can cause cerebral edema and may result in hemorrhagic stroke. Classic signs of hyperperfusion syndrome are a headache on the same side as the revascularized carotid artery and the onset of focal motor seizures. Strict control of postoperative blood pressure is an important aspect of the management of patients undergoing endarterectomy.

Classic Case

A 76-year-old man with coronary artery disease and hypertension presents to his internist after an episode loss of vision in his right eye. He describes the event as occurring suddenly with no preceding symptoms and resolving after a few minutes. He denies any prior similar events or other neurologic symptoms. Auscultation over the right neck reveals a carotid bruit. A duplex ultrasound is ordered and demonstrates an 80 % stenosis of the right carotid artery. The patient is started on aspirin and a statin, and is counseled to under carotid endarterectomy to lower his chances of a future stroke. A cardiac evaluation reveals no prohibitive risk for surgery. A CT angiogram is obtained for operative planning.

The patient undergoes a right carotid endarterectomy under general anesthesia. EEG monitoring is used to monitor his neurologic status and no shunt is employed. The case is uneventful and upon waking from anesthesia his speech and motor activities are normal. In the postoperative period the patient experiences labile blood pressures and requires close hypertensive control. The patient recovers without further incident and is discharged home.

OR Questions

1. Does the pitch of a carotid bruit correlate with the degree of stenosis?
   No. While a carotid bruit is a general indicator of the presence of atherosclerotic disease, its sound does not correlate with severity of stenosis.
2. What structures are contained within the carotid sheath?
   The carotid artery, internal jugular vein, vagus nerve, and deep cervical lymph nodes.
3. Injury to the hypoglossal nerve causes what defect?
   Tongue deviation toward the injured nerve.
4. Where is the carotid bulb and what is its function?
   The carotid sinus, or bulb, is a dilatation of the carotid artery at the level of the bifurcation. This structure contains special baroreceptors that are innervated by branches of the glossopharyngeal nerve and are involved in maintenance of normal blood pressure. Physical stimulation of the carotid bulb during endarterectomy can cause reflexive hypotension.
5. In a patient with who presents with an acute stroke and is found to have significant carotid stenosis, when is the preferred timing of surgical intervention?
   Carotid endarterectomy should be performed approximately 2 weeks after the neurologic event, once the symptoms have plateaued.
6. What is the first branch of the external carotid artery?
   Superior thyroid artery.
7. If the carotid artery is found to have 100 % stenosis (i.e., complete occlusion), should a CEA be performed?
   No, revascularization after complete occlusion of the carotid consists of extra-to-intracranial carotid bypass; it is associ-

ated with high complication rates and has not been shown to be more efficient in preventing subsequent strokes compared to best medical treatment.

Carotid Endarterectomy

Pathophysiology
- Atherosclerotic plaque develops at the common carotid artery bifurcation
- Symptoms may be caused either by plaque emboli or low flow through stenotic vessel
- Degree of stenosis can be evaluated by duplex ultrasound, angiography, MRA, or CTA

Symptoms
- Transient ischemic attack
- Ischemic stroke
- Amaurosis fugax: transient monocular blindness caused by an embolus to the ophthalmic artery
- Vertigo and syncope are not generally symptoms of carotid disease

Indications
- Symptomatic patients: endarterectomy recommended for patients with >70 % stenosis, and in select patients with >50 % stenosis
- Asymptomatic patients: less evidence for benefit, some recommend non-operative therapy only, others recommend CEA for men with >60 % stenosis

Non-operative management
- Antiplatelet agents / aspirin
- Cholesterol lowering agents
- Antihypertensives
- Carotid artery stenting: generally reserved for patients considered too high risk for endarterectomy, or for those with re-stenosis following prior CEA

Technique
- General or local anesthesia
- Incision along the sternocleidomastoid muscle
- Proximal and distal vascular control obtained
- Systemic heparinization
- Longitudinal arteriotomy
- Placement of shunt, per surgeon preference
- Atherosclerotic plaque is dissected off the vessel wall
- Carotid artery is flushed
- A patch of vein or prosthetic material used to close the carotid without narrowing

Peri-op orders
- Pre-operative aspirin
- Pre-incision antibiotics
- Intra-op heparinization
- Serial neurologic exams
- Blood pressure monitoring
- Advance diet as tolerated

Complications
- Acute myocardial infarction
- Post-operative stroke
- Neck hematoma
- Hyperperfusion syndrome
- Cranial nerve injury
- Carotid artery restenosis

Suggested Reading

Rockman CB, Jacobowitz GR. Carotid endarterectomy with shunt. In: Fischer JE, Jones DB, Pomposelli FB, Upchurch GR, Klimberg VS, Schwaitzberg SD, Bland KI, editors. Fischer's mastery of surgery. 6th ed. Philadelphia: Lippincott Williams & Wilkins; 2012.

29
Abdominal Aortic Aneurysm Repair

Introduction

An **abdominal aortic aneurysm** (AAA) is defined as a focal dilation of the aorta beyond a diameter of 3.0 cm. The causes of aneurysmal degeneration of the aorta are multifactorial, and likely involve a combination of risk factors that lead to a loss of vascular structural proteins and wall strength. Both age and gender are important predisposing factors, as demonstrated by the observation that the rate of AAA rises sharply after age 60, and men develop aortic aneurysms more frequently than women. The greatest acquired risk factor for both the onset and growth of an AAA is smoking. Poorly controlled hypertension also contributes to aneurysm formation and growth.

Most AAAs develop in the region between the renal arteries and the aortic bifurcation, and are accordingly termed **infrarenal aortic aneurysms** (Fig. 29.1). The reason that aneurysms form in this location is likely related to the changes in fluid dynamics and increased wall pressures that occur as the aorta bifurcates into the iliac arteries. Structural differences and a lower collagen to elastin ratio in the abdominal aortic wall as compared to thoracic aorta, may also play a role. As an aneurysm progresses, it can expand proximally above the level of the renal arteries, as well as distally to cause aneurismal dilatation of the iliac arteries.

U. Sarpel, *Surgery: An Introductory Guide*,
DOI 10.1007/978-1-4939-0903-2_29,
© Springer Science+Business Media New York 2014

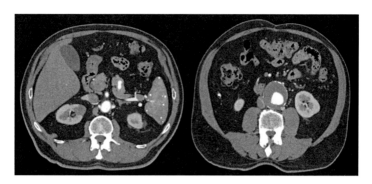

FIG. 29.1 Axial CT images of a patient with a normal caliber aorta at the level of the renal arteries and a 5.3 cm aneurysm with mural thrombus in the infrarenal aorta

Most patients with an AAA are asymptomatic, and the aneurysm is only detected as an incidental finding on imaging studies performed for other purposes. Occasionally, a pulsatile mass is detected on routine physical examination. AAA can also present with lower extremity ischemia due to distal embolization of atherosclerotic debris from the aneurysm sac. When symptoms of AAA do occur, patients may present with vague abdominal or back pain, presumably from compression of nearby structures by the enlarging aneurysm sac. The presence of severe back pain may be an ominous sign of impeding rupture. However, since AAAs are typically asymptomatic, individuals considered at high risk should be enrolled in screening programs that use abdominal ultrasounds to measure aortic diameter.

The natural history of AAAs is of a progressive increase in size and eventual **rupture** (Fig. 29.2). There are currently no treatments to reverse the course of an AAA, but growth of the aneurysm can be slowed with exercise, control of blood pressure, and smoking cessation. Once a patient has been diagnosed with an aneurysm, close surveillance is necessary to follow its diameter. Expansion rates vary between individuals, and the growth of an aneurysm typically accelerates as the diameter becomes increasingly wide. The risk for

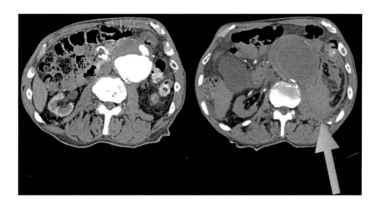

F<small>IG</small>. 29.2 Axial CT image demonstrating a 7.5 cm AAA in a patient who was not a surgical candidate. The patient later presented with back pain and CT images revealed a contained rupture of the aneurysm; note the retroperitoneal extravasation of blood (*arrow*)

rupture rises markedly at aneurysm diameters greater than 5.5 cm. As a result, surgical repair is generally advised when aneurysm size approaches this size, or if an aneurysm is noted to be expanding rapidly on serial imaging.

Intervention prior to rupture is critical since – once rupture occurs – only about half of patients survive long enough to reach a medical facility. Free rupture of an AAA with intraperitoneal hemorrhage produces profound hemodynamic instability and is rapidly fatal. However, rupture of the posterior aortic wall may be initially contained within the retroperitoneum, allowing the opportunity for treatment. Rupture of an AAA is said to produce a triad of severe acute pain, a pulsatile abdominal mass, and hypotension, although this classic presentation is only seen in about half of patients.

Any patient seen in the emergency room with a suspicion of a ruptured AAA must be evaluated immediately. Physical examination should include assessment of the palpation of the abdomen in the region between the xiphoid and umbilicus, to identify a pulsatile mass. If the patient has a contained rupture, the associated retroperitoneal hematoma may track to the skin to produce a visible ecchymosis in the mid-back

(**Grey-Turner sign**) or in the periumbilical region (**Cullen's sign**). Despite the fact that patients with a ruptured AAA will be hypotensive, fluid restriction should be restricted, since any added intravascular volume may convert a contained rupture into a free rupture.

In a hemodynamically unstable patient, with a known history of an AAA, who presents with signs of rupture, imaging is not required to confirm the diagnosis. In this scenario, patients who are candidates for surgical repair should be taken straight to the operating room without any preceding imaging study. In patients with no history of an AAA, a rapid non-contrast CT scan should be obtained to confirm the presence of an aneurysm.

Abdominal aortic aneurysms can be repaired by an open surgical approach or via **endovascular aneurysm repair** (**EVAR**). In open surgery, the aneurismal portion of the aorta is replaced with a synthetic graft. The endovascular approach involves the use of an **endograft**, which is deployed within the aneurismal aorta from a remote site, typically the femoral artery. Fixation of the endovascular device is achieved against the normal (non-dilated) segment of the aortic wall proximally just below the renal arteries, and distally in each of the iliac arteries distally. The device creates a seal, excluding the aneurysm sac from blood flow, and thereby preventing expansion of the AAA.

The pros and cons of the open versus endovascular approach should be considered on a case-by-case basis.

However, not all patients are candidates for both types of repair. One consideration in selecting the approach is that open AAA repair must be performed under general anesthesia, while EVAR can be performed with local anesthesia and sedation. Contraindications to open repair of an AAA include extensive intra-abdominal adhesions, morbid obesity, and major cardiac or pulmonary comorbidities.

By contrast, contraindications for endovascular repair are largely centered on technical aspects of the aneurysm's shape and location. In order to successfully exclude blood flow into the aneurysm sac, the endograft must provide an adequate seal where it contacts the arterial wall. A short neck between the AAA and the renal arteries is therefore a relative contraindication to endovascular repair. In addition, features such as sharp angulation of the aorta or iliac arteries can interfere with proper positioning and fixation of the device. Prior to AAA repair, CT or MR angiography is used to evaluate the anatomic features of the aneurysm that may affect the approach to repair. Finally, since endograft size and shape must be carefully customized for each patient's specific anatomy, emergent repair of a ruptured AAA via the endovascular approach is only possible in centers where a wide selection of variously sized endografts is immediately available. Overall endovascular repair is associated with less mortality and morbidity but requires lifelong surveillance of the endograft with CT angiography. Because of the higher perioperative survival, endovascular repair is emerging as the preferable technique in patients undergoing elective repair who have suitable anatomy.

Surgical Technique

Open AAA repair can be performed through a standard midline laparotomy, or via a posterior retroperitoneal approach. The retroperitoneal method is less commonly performed, but may be used to avoid adhesions associated with prior intraabdominal operations or in cases of inflammatory AAA. The anterior, transabdominal approach is the most common method of open repair, and will be described below. This is also the preferred approach in the setting of a ruptured AAA, since clamping of the aorta can be accomplished rapidly upon entering the abdomen.

Once the abdomen has been accessed, the bowel is reflected away to expose the retroperitoneum and the great vessels. The retroperitoneum is incised, the third and fourth portions of the duodenum are mobilized, and the surrounding tissues are gently dissected away to expose the aorta from the **renal arteries** down to the **common iliac arteries** (Fig. 29.3).

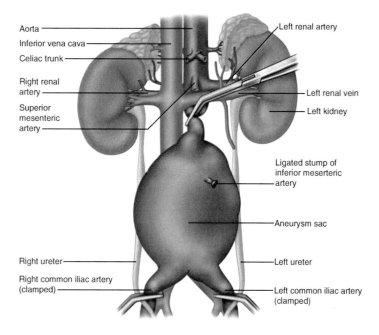

FIG. 29.3 Surgical anatomy during open abdominal aortic aneurysm repair: aorta, inferior vena cava, right and left renal arteries, left renal vein, right and left common iliac arteries, right and left ureters, and inferior mesenteric artery

The **inferior mesenteric artery** (IMA), which arises at the level of the aneurysmal aorta, is ligated. In most individuals, adequate blood supply to the left colon is maintained even with ligation of the inferior mesenteric artery, through collateral supply via the **marginal artery of Drummond**. However, the inferior mesenteric artery should be reimplanted at the completion of the case if there is any question of colonic ischemia.

After confirming the anatomy of the aneurysm and the plan for repair, systemic heparin is administered to reduce the risk of arterial thrombosis during clamping. Vascular control of the aneurysm is then obtained by clamping first the common iliac arteries, followed by the aorta just below the renal arteries. Once the clamps are in place, the aorta is opened longitudinally. Thrombus within the aneurysm sac is evacuated and retrograde bleeding from the lumbar arteries is controlled with suture ligation. The aortic cuff is then prepared by dividing the anterior wall of the aorta transversely for about half the circumference. The posterior wall of the aorta is typically left intact, although technique can vary. The distal aorta (or bilateral iliac arteries depending on the extent of the AAA) is prepared in the same manner.

The aorta is then reconstructed using a synthetic graft. The proximal and distal anastomoses are performed using a nonabsorbable suture. Once the repair is complete, the clamps are serially removed to reestablish blood flow. Finally the native aortic wall is then closed over the graft, in order to prevent contact of the prosthetic graft material with adjacent bowel.

After completion of the anastomosis, pulses in the femoral arteries as well as in the feet should be assessed to confirm the adequacy of distal blood flow. Finally, the descending colon should once again be inspected for the presence of ischemia to determine if the inferior mesenteric artery requires reimplantation.

For endovascular repair of an AAA, the first step is the preoperative selection of appropriately shaped and sized graft components, as determined by the patient's angiogram. In most cases, a main graft device is used to span the body of the aneurysm, and one or two additional components are used to extend into each of the iliac arteries. Bilateral femoral artery access is required for placement of each limb of the stent graft, and this approach can be via open groin incisions or percutaneous puncture. Once vascular access is established, an angiogram is obtained and the landmarks for positioning the endograft are determined. The collapsed stent graft loaded on the delivery device is introduced through the common femoral artery and positioned within the aorta, taking care to correctly align the opening for the contralateral limb and maintain patency of the renal arteries. Once the main graft has been deployed, the second limb is introduced via the opposite femoral artery. This component is then

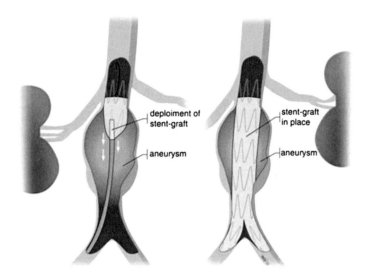

FIG. 29.4 Endovascular repair of an infrarenal abdominal aortic aneurysm with a bifurcated stent graft. [Reprinted Santos ICT, Sepulveda AT, Viana JC, et al. Improving Post-EVAR Surveillance with a Smart Stent-Graft. In: Jorge RMN, Tavares JMRS, Barbosa MP, Slade AP, (eds). Technologies for Medical Sciences. Netherlands: Springer Verlag; 2012:267-289. With permission from Springer Verlag]

deployed, taking care to overlap with the primary stent. The process is repeated for the ipsilateral iliac limb, as needed (Fig. 29.4). A balloon is then used to fully expand the stents and ensure a tight seal with the vessel wall. Finally, a completion angiogram is obtained to confirm patency of the renal arteries, and to ensure that exclusion of blood flow from the aneurysm sac has been achieved (Fig. 29.5).

Complications

While some complications of AAA repair apply to both open and endovascular techniques, others are specific to the type of approach used. **Lower extremity ischemia** may occur with

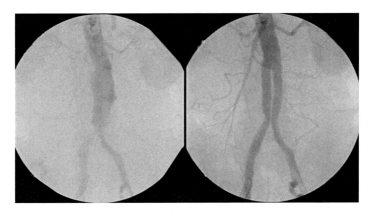

F<small>IG</small>. 29.5 Angiogram of the patient in Fig. 29.1, before and after endovascular aneurysm repair

either method, as a result of distal embolization, arterial dissection, or a technical problem or clot at the distal graft site. Pulses of the lower extremity should always be documented at the completion of the case, and then followed closely in the postoperative period. If a sudden loss of pulse occurs in the immediate postoperative period, the patient should be taken back to the operating room, and may require thrombectomy and/or operative revision of the iliac anastomosis.

Cardiac events, such as **acute myocardial infarction**, are the most frequent serious complication of AAA repair, whether open or endovascular, and are the most common cause of postoperative death. Patient selection for AAA repair must therefore include careful risk stratification of patient comorbidities and preoperative optimization of cardiac status.

Some degree of **renal dysfunction** is not unusual following AAA repair. Direct ischemia can occur from occlusion of the renal arteries by the endograft at EVAR, or during open repair if suprarenal clamping of the aorta is performed. **Contrast-induced nephropathy** can be seen after EVAR, owing to the amounts of contrast used for the intraoperative angiograms. In most instances, postoperative renal dysfunction is transient and resolves with fluid hydration.

Colonic ischemia can occur if the descending colon is dependent on the IMA for adequate perfusion, and this vessel is ligated at surgery. Patients with colonic ischemia may be asymptomatic, or may present with left lower quadrant abdominal pain, bloody diarrhea, or rising lactate levels. Fortunately in most patients, the ischemia is limited to the colonic mucosa and will resolve with supportive care alone. If the ischemic insult is severe however, full-thickness necrosis can develop, requiring surgical resection of the affected segment of bowel.

Graft infection is a rare but serious and usually late complication of AAA repair. Once a foreign body has been contaminated with bacteria, antibiotics alone are unlikely to result in long-term clearance of the infection. Some cases may require extra-anatomical vascular bypass and explantation of the graft material, which can be an extremely morbid procedure. Pre-incision antibiotics are used to decrease this possibility of infection.

Aortoenteric fistula is one of the most devastating complications of aortic surgery. Mechanical erosion of the prosthetic graft into the adjacent duodenum can result in dramatic arterial bleeding into the lumen of the GI tract. This condition classically manifests with a brief, self-limited episode of hematemesis, known as a **sentinel bleed**. Treatment involves urgent excision of the graft and extra-anatomic revascularization. If the sentinel bleed is not recognized, the condition invariably progresses to exsanguinating hemorrhage.

An **endoleak** refers to the presence of persistent blood flow into the aneurysm sac following EVAR (Fig. 29.6). Five types of endoleak have been described; Type 1 is an incompetent seal at the proximal or distal attachment sites, Type 2 consists of retrograde flow into the sac from patent lumbar arteries or IMA; Type 3 is a leak between endograft components; and Type 4 is a leak due to porosity of the graft material and is self-limited (Fig. 29.7). Finally a Type 5 endoleak, or endotension, refers to leak not well identified but associated

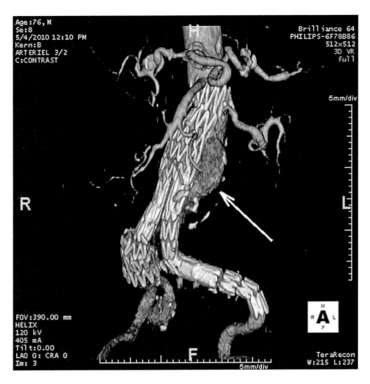

FIG. 29.6 3D-CT image of a patient following endovascular AAA repair, demonstrating persistent flow into the aneurysm sac as a result of an endoleak. [Reprinted from Kpodonu J, Haulon S, Midulla M. Complications in Endoaortic Surgery: Endoleaks After Endovascular Repair of the Abdominal Aorta. In: Kpodonu J, Haulon S (eds). Atlas of Advanced Endoaortic Surgery. London, UK: Springer Verlag; 2013:135-151. With permission from Springer Verlag]

with sac growth on surveillance imaging. Importantly, Types 1, 3, and 5 are associated with a continued risk for aneurysm expansion or rupture. One of the relative disadvantages of EVAR is that patients must be enrolled in long-term imaging surveillance to detect the development of an endoleak.

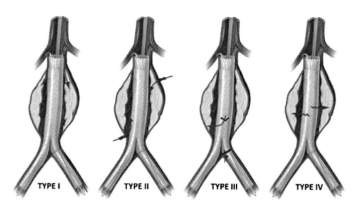

FIG. 29.7 Types of endoleak. [Reprinted from Figueroa CA, Zarins CK. Computational analysis of displacement forces acting on endografts used to treat aortic aneurysms. In: McGloughlin T, editor. Biomechanics and mechanobiology of aneurysms. Heidelberg: Springer Verlag; 2011. p. 221-46. With permission from Springer Verlag]

Classic Case

A 73-year-old man is brought into the emergency room with a complaint of sudden, severe lower back pain. He reports a history of hypertension and smoking, but has not seen a doctor in many years. On examination he is found to be hypotensive to 87/55 mmHg. A ruptured AAA is suspected, but a pulsatile mass cannot be appreciated on palpation of the abdomen. An urgent non-contrast CT scan is performed and demonstrates a 6.5 cm infrarenal aortic aneurysm with a contained retroperitoneal rupture. The patient is taken emergently to the operating room for open repair. The anesthesiology team places large-bore IVs and an arterial line, and orders several units of packed red blood cells.

A midline laparotomy is performed and rapid proximal control of the aorta is achieved by clamping the supraceliac aorta. As soon as vascular control is obtained, the patient is resuscitated, and the clamp is moved down to the infrarenal aorta to allow reperfusion of the kidneys. A standard AAA repair is then performed, and the patient is transferred to the SICU after completion of surgery.

On postoperative day #2 the patient has a bloody, loose bowel movement. His hemodynamic parameters and white blood cell count are all within normal limits, but his lactate is mildly elevated at 3.5 mmol/L. A sigmoidoscopy is performed and demonstrates that the mucosa of the descending colon is pale with areas of petechial bleeding, consistent with colonic ischemia. The patient is placed on bowel rest, and supportive care with intravenous fluids and empiric broad spectrum antibiotics are provided. Over the next 2 days, the patient has no further episodes of bloody bowel movements and is restarted on an oral diet.

OR Questions

1. What genetic disorder is associated with higher rates of AAA?
   Marfan syndrome is an autosomal dominant condition caused by a mutation in the gene that encodes for the protein fibrillin, an integral component of connective tissue. Mutations in this gene result in a wide spectrum of connective tissue disorders, including higher rates of aneurysm formation.

2. Can an angiogram be used to measure the size of an aneurysm?
   No, an angiogram only demonstrates the diameter of the patent lumen. The size of an aneurysm is the total cross-sectional diameter of the entire aneurysm sac, including any mural thrombus. (Compare Figures 29.1 and 29.5).

3. Are multiple vascular aneurysms a common occurrence?
   Yes, patients with a popliteal or a femoral artery aneurysm frequently have a concurrent abdominal aortic aneurysm, and should be screened accordingly.

4. During open AAA repair, what is the implication of vigorous back-bleeding from the stump of the inferior mesenteric artery?
   Brisk, pulsatile bleeding from the IMA stump indicates the presence of adequate collateral blood flow from the SMA, and implies that reimplantation into the aortic graft is not necessary.

5. What test can be performed to assess for full-thickness colonic ischemia?
A sigmoidoscopy only visualizes the mucosa of the bowel. If there is concern for full-thickness ischemia, a diagnostic laparoscopy should be performed to inspect the serosal aspect of the colon.

Abdominal Aortic Aneurysm Repair

Pathophysiology
- Smoking, age >60, male gender, and hypertension are major risk factors
- Increasing diameter of the aneurysm is associated with rupture, as described by the Law of Laplace

Indication
- Normal aortic diameter is 1.5-3 cm
- Ultrasound is used to monitor the growth of a known aneurysm
- Repair recommended once >5.5 cm, or if rapid growth detected

Symptoms
- Intact aneurysms are generally asymptomatic
- Typically found incidentally on imaging, or by a palpation of pulsatile abdominal mass
- Free rupture causes hemorrhagic shock and is rapidly fatal
- Contained rupture may present with sudden lower back or abdominal pain and hypotension

Technique: Open repair
- Midline laparotomy
- Retroperitoneum is incised and aorta exposed
- Ligation of IMA (may be reimplanted if necessary)
- Systemic heparinization
- Clamping of bilateral iliac arteries, then infrarenal aorta
- Aneurysm sac is opened and thrombus is evacuated
- Proximal and distal cuffs are prepared
- Synthetic graft is sewn into place
- Native aorta is closed over the graft

Technique: Endovascular repair (EVAR)
- Bilateral femoral artery access established
- Angiogram obtained and landmarks confirmed
- Systemic heparinization
- Main device is introduced through the common femoral artery, positioned in aorta, and deployed
- Contralateral and ipsilateral iliac limbs are deployed, overlapping with main stent
- Balloon angioplasty
- Completion angiogram

Peri-op orders
- Pre-incision antibiotics
- Intra-operative heparinization
- Post-op pulse exam
- Hemodynamic monitoring
- Advance diet as tolerated

Complications
- Lower extremity ischemia
- Renal ischemia or contrast nephropathy
- Left colonic ischemia
- Aortoenteric fistula
- Endoleak: persistent flow of blood into the aneurysm sac following EVAR

Suggested Reading

Schermerhorn ML, Cronenwett JL. Natural history and decision making for abdominal aortic aneurysms. In: Zelenock GB, Huber TS, Messina LM, Lumsden AB, Moneta GL, editors. Mastery of vascular and endovascular surgery: an illustrated review. 1st ed. Philadelphia: Lippincott Williams & Wilkins; 2006.

30
Vascular Bypass

Introduction

Peripheral arterial disease (PAD) describes the condition in which atherosclerotic plaques deposit in the vessels of the extremities, usually the legs (Fig. 30.1). Predictably, the risk factors for PAD include smoking, hypertension, diabetes, and hyperlipidemia, and this condition typically coexists with coronary artery disease. Many patients with PAD are asymptomatic, however, some will develop intermittent pain in the buttock, thigh, or calf muscles, known as claudication. There are many causes of leg pain unrelated to PAD, therefore it is important to be specific when eliciting potential symptoms. In order to qualify as true **claudication**, the leg pain must involve a muscle group, be reproducibly caused by exertion, and relieved with rest. The pathophysiology of claudication is analogous to angina; pain occurs when the muscles of the leg experience ischemia because their metabolic needs exceed the inflow of arterial blood. The site of pain usually correlates with the level of disease: calf claudication is usually caused by disease in the superficial femoral artery, where as thigh or buttock claudication indicates more proximal occlusion, typically at the iliac artery.

As PAD progresses, the arterial supply to the lower extremities may become insufficient to maintain even the baseline metabolic needs of the foot, resulting in **rest pain**. Patients with rest pain classically dangle their affected leg off

U. Sarpel, *Surgery: An Introductory Guide*,
DOI 10.1007/978-1-4939-0903-2_30,
© Springer Science+Business Media New York 2014

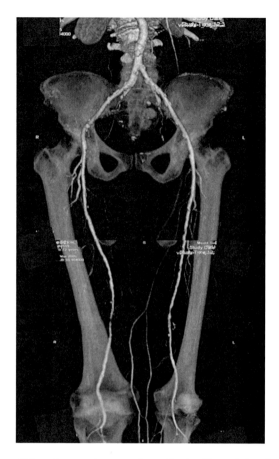

FIG. 30.1 CT angiogram images of a patient with peripheral arterial disease demonstrating narrowing of bilateral superficial femoral arteries

the side of the bed, because the gravity-induced increase in blood flow to the foot helps to relieve the pain. Another sign of advanced PAD is a non-healing **ischemic ulcer** of the foot. These ulcers are typically located on the lateral aspect of the ankle or the toes. This distribution is distinct from ulcers caused by venous stasis, which are usually found on the medial aspect of the ankle. Ultimately, peripheral arterial disease can lead to frank gangrene of the toes.

Any patient suspected of having PAD should undergo a complete history and physical, including a bilateral pulse examination with palpation of the femoral, popliteal, posterior tibial, and dorsalis pedis pulses. Diminished or absent pulses should be noted, and a Doppler device can be used to search for signal in sites where pulses are not palpable. The point of transition from normal to absent pulses usually indicates the level of vascular stenosis.

The **ankle-brachial index** (ABI) is a way to quantify the degree of decreased blood flow to the extremities. The ABI is a ratio of the blood pressure at the level of the ankle over that in the arm (Fig. 30.2). An ABI of 1 means that the blood pressure in the extremities is equal to the systemic blood pressure and therefore no vascular disease is present. An ABI less than 0.9 is abnormal and suggests the presence of peripheral arterial disease. An ABI less than 0.8 is indicative of moderate PAD, and an ABI less than 0.4 indicates severe PAD, usually associated with ischemic ulcers or gangrene.

It is important to note that ABI measurements in diabetics are typically unreliable. The calcifications of peripheral vessels that occur in this disease cause them to be less compressible, leading to falsely normal ABIs, or values greater than 1. In such patients, or toe pressures or **pulse volume recordings** of the leg, which are not affected by calcifications, can be used to diagnose the presence of PAD (Fig. 30.3).

In the absence of devitalized tissue, PAD should be treated first with lifestyle modifications and pharmacologic therapy. Smoking cessation should be strongly recommended. Antiplatelet therapy and medications for cholesterol reduction are also prescribed. In patients with claudication, **exercise therapy** can be used for symptom reduction. Patients are instructed to ambulate until claudication occurs, and then to continue walking for several more minutes before resting. This exercise-rest cycle is repeated several times per session. These periods of ischemia are thought to induce muscle remodeling, ultimately allowing a patient to ambulate a greater distance before claudication occurs. Exercise therapy requires a motivated patient since it must be performed several times a week for 1–2 months before the benefits become evident.

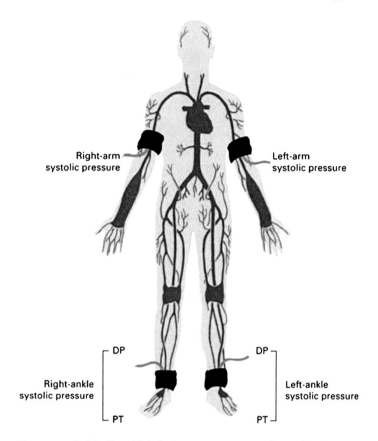

FIG. 30.2 Ankle-Brachial Index measurement [Reprinted from Petznick AM, Shubrook JH. Treatment of specific macrovascular beds in patients with diabetes mellitus. Osteopathic Medicine and Primary Care 2010; 4:5. With permission from BioMed Central Ltd]

The presence of claudication is not in itself an indication for surgery. Intervention should be strictly reserved for those patients with disabling claudication, rest pain, non-healing ischemic ulcers, or gangrene. The reason for reserving surgical treatment until clearly indicated is that revascularization procedures for PAD have a limited period of patency of 5–10

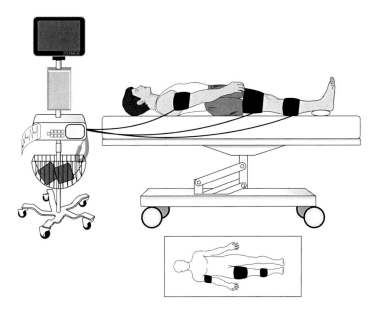

F<small>IG</small>. 30.3 Pulse volume recordings [Reprinted from Raines JK, Almeida JI. Pulse Volume Recording in the Diagnosis of Peripheral Vascular Disease. In: AbuRahma AF, Bandyk DF (eds). Noninvasive Vascular Diagnosis: A Practical Guide to Therapy. London, UK: Springer Verlag; 2013: 303-310. With permission from Springer Verlag]

years. Performing bypass prematurely both exposes the patient to unnecessary surgical risk, and limits the surgical options for treatment of recurrent disease.

Patients with indications for intervention should be evaluated with CT angiography to delineate the arterial anatomy and to assess which of the options are most appropriate. Revascularization procedures for PAD include **endovascular angioplasty/stenting**, **endarterectomy**, **vascular bypass**, or possibly **amputation**. Angioplasty or stenting is suitable for patients with relatively focal flow-limiting lesions (Fig. 30.4). Vascular bypass may be an option for patients with more extensive segments of disease, but requires certain anatomic

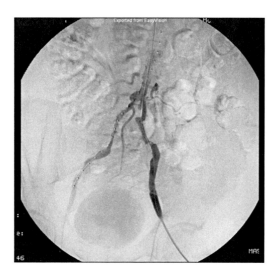

Fɪɢ. 30.4 Intraoperative angiogram image of a patient with bilateral aortoiliac occlusive disease undergoing iliac stenting

features including adequate arterial inflow and a relatively disease-free target vessel (Fig. 30.5). Occasionally, a combination of these approaches can be used, such as angioplasty of a proximal vessel in order to improve the arterial inflow for a downstream vascular bypass.

Several types of vascular bypass exist, depending on the area of disease that is being bypassed. Commonly performed types of vascular bypass include aortobifemoral bypass, iliofemoral bypass (Fig. 30.6), femoro-femoral bybass, femoropopliteal bypass, and distal bypasses to the tibial or pedal vessels. Either autologous vein or a synthetic graft may be used as the conduit. The ipsilateral or contralateral greater saphenous vein is generally the preferred conduit, however since PAD patients are often also cardiac surgery patients, the saphenous may have been previously harvested for coronary artery bypass grafting. In this situation, the basilic or cephalic veins of the arm can be used as an alternative.

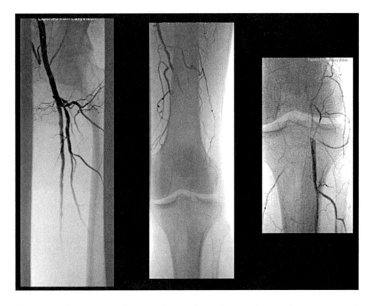

FIG. 30.5 Intraoperative angiography of a patient who presented with left toe gangrene, demonstrating a diseased superficial femoral artery with distal occlusion and reconstitution of the popliteal artery. The patient underwent a superficial femoral artery to below-knee popliteal bypass

Vein mapping by ultrasound is useful to identify the most suitable veins prior to surgery.

Amputations are generally the last resort for patients with gangrene or non-healing wounds where revascularization is not feasible or beneficial. The level of amputation required is determined by the distribution of devitalized tissue as well as by the robustness of the underlying arterial supply. For example, in a patient with toe gangrene, a single digit amputation is unlikely to heal if there is not sufficient arterial supply to the remaining foot. In this patient, a more proximal amputation may be required to ensure healing of the stump. Progressively higher levels of amputation are a **transmetatarsal amputation**, a **below-knee amputation**, and an **above-knee amputation**.

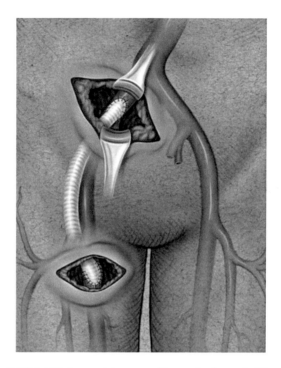

FIG. 30.6 Right iliofemoral bypass with synthetic graft. [Reprinted from Kpodonu J. Endovascular Management of a Thoracic Aortic Aneurysm Using a Retroperitoneal Conduit. In: Kpodonu J (ed). Manual of Thoracic Endoaortic Surgery. London, UK: Springer Verlag; 2010: 335-342. With permission from Springer Verlag]

Surgical Technique

Although several types of vascular bypass exist, a femoral to below-knee popliteal bypass is described as a representative example. The procedure begins with the groin incision where the common **femoral, deep femoral, and superficial femoral arteries** are dissected out (Fig. 30.7). Vascular control is obtained by placing vessel loops around these structures. Next a skin incision is made along the medial aspect of the

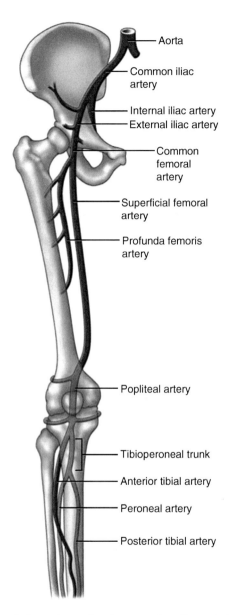

FIG. 30.7 Surgical anatomy for lower extremity arterial bypass: aorta, common iliac artery, external iliac artery, internal iliac artery, common femoral artery, superficial femoral artery, profunda femoris artery, popliteal artery, anterior tibial artery, tibioperoneal trunk, peroneal artery, and posterior tibial artery

knee, extending onto the calf. The popliteal space is entered and control is obtained of the distal **popliteal artery**. The **saphenous vein** harvest is performed next. The proximal portion of the vein is ligated in the groin and the distal portion is ligated in medial aspect of the knee. Typically, several skip incisions are made down the thigh, which allows the vein to be excised while sparing the patient a long incision. The vein is harvested, taking care to carefully tie off all branches. The vein is then flushed with heparin to check for any leaks. Since the saphenous vein contains several one-way valves, it is typically anastomosed in reversed position to allow for unimpeded flow. Alternatively, a long valvulotome can be used to disrupt the venous valves and allow anterograde flow.

Next, a tunnel is created beneath the sartorius muscle connecting the groin and popliteal incisions. The vein or synthetic graft is passed through the tunnel and brought to lie into position. Systemic heparinization is administered and the femoral artery is clamped. The femoral arteriotomy is made, and the proximal anastomosis is performed using a fine, nonabsorbable suture. The distal anastomosis is performed next, using a similar technique. The vessels are unclamped and arterial flow is reestablished. A completion angiogram is performed to confirm adequate flow, and the distal pulses are carefully assessed. The wounds are closed in layers.

Complications

Acute myocardial infarction is a common cause of postoperative morbidity following vascular bypass since all patients with PAD also have some degree of coronary artery disease. As a result, patients being considered for bypass surgery should first undergo a thorough cardiac assessment and optimization of cardiac function.

Graft infection after vascular bypass is a rare, but serious complication of the use of a synthetic conduit. Infection can occur either as a result of direct contamination of the graft, or from seeding due to a systemic bacteremia. Patients typically present with fever and signs of local wound infection, including erythema, edema, and wound discharge. Surgical excision of the prosthesis is invariably required because antibiotics alone are insufficient to eradicate an infectious process when a foreign body is present.

Graft occlusion can be an acute or chronic complication of bypass. In the immediate postoperative period, graft occlusion may be due to technical issues with the graft or from thrombosis. Close monitoring of the distal pulse is necessary to detect graft occlusion in a timely fashion. Once graft occlusion has been diagnosed, initiation of anticoagulation is imperative to halt thrombus propagation. Immediate re-exploration is usually indicated to evacuate clot and to assess for technical problems such as kinking of the conduit or narrowing of the anastomosis. Late graft failure is usually attributable to **intimal hyperplasia** or recurrent atherosclerosis. Unfortunately, there are few therapeutic options for late graft failure; endovascular intervention or surgical revision is usually required.

Classic Case

A 74-year-old man, who is an active smoker and has coronary artery disease, presents to his primary care doctor with a complaint of left calf pain. The pain occurs after he walks about two blocks, and resolves with rest. A pulse exam demonstrates bilateral palpable femoral pulses. The right dorsalis pedis pulse is palpable, but the left can only be detected with a Doppler. He has no evidence of gangrene or non-healing wounds. The ABI is 0.8 on the right, and 0.5 on the left. The patient is started on aspirin and a statin, and advised to stop smoking. He is also enrolled in exercise therapy.

One year later, the patient returns with increasing left foot pain, which is now constant and present even at rest. On examination the left foot is ruborous. He admits poor compliance with the recommended lifestyle modifications. He is referred to a vascular surgeon for evaluation of his critical limb ischemia. A CT angiogram demonstrates occlusion of a long segment of the left superficial femoral artery, with reconstitution at the level of the popliteal artery, and normal three-vessel run-off. The profunda femoris artery has multiple stenoses. He has a normal echocardiogram and stress test and is cleared for surgery. A left femoropopliteal bypass using a reversed saphenous vein graft is performed. Postoperatively the patient's pulses are closely monitored. He has an eventful recovery and is ultimately discharged home.

OR Questions

1. What are the layers of the arterial wall?
   The layers from outside, inward are the adventitia, the media, and the intima.
2. What is Leriche syndrome?
   The triad of buttock claudication, diminished femoral pulses, and erectile dysfunction is known as Leriche syndrome. This condition generally indicates the presence of aortoiliac occlusive disease.
3. Is gangrene of the toe a surgical emergency?
   Dry gangrene is not an emergency, however wet gangrene represents infected tissue and a guillotine amputation should be performed urgently.
4. Why are synthetic conduits avoided for below-knee bypasses?
   Repeated bending of the graft at the knee joint can lead to inferior patency rates compared to autologous conduits.
5. What is an extra-anatomic bypass and when is it used?
   An extra-anatomic bypass consists of an arterial bypass with a synthetic graft that does not follow the normal anatomic pathway. Examples of such bypasses are the femoro-femoral bypass, axillo-femoral bypass, and carotid-subclavian bypass.

The conduits are used only in cases of prior graft infection when it is necessary to avoid areas with infected tissue, or when no other revascularization options exist due to physiologic or anatomic reasons.

Vascular Bypass

Pathophysiology
- Risk factors: cigarette smoking, diabetes, hypertension, high cholesterol
- Atherosclerotic plaques develop over time, leading to narrowing of the vessel
- Claudication: reproducible pain caused by exercise and relieved with rest, occurs as a result of ischemia

Evaluation
- Pulse exam
- Ankle brachial index: blood pressure is measured at the ankle and divided by the brachial artery pressure
- Pulse volume recordings
- CT angiography
- Invasive angiography

Indications for intervention
- Disabling claudication
- Non-healing ulcer
- Gangrene
- Rest pain

Technique
- Angiography to confirm anatomy
- Exposure of inflow vessel with proximal and distal vascular control
- Exposure of outflow vessel with proximal and distal vascular control
- Vein harvest, if applicable
- Systemic heparinization
- Arteriotomy of inflow vessel
- Proximal anastomosis
- Tunneling of graft to distal site
- Distal anastomosis
- Angiography to confirm flow
- Pulse exam

Non-operative management
- Smoking cessation is the most important intervention
- Exercise induces angiogenesis in affected muscle group and improves claudication
- Statin therapy
- Aspirin therapy

Peri-op orders
- Pre-incision antibiotics
- Intra-op systemic heparinization
- Post-op pulse exam monitoring
- Post-operative anticoagulation
- Advance diet as tolerated

Complications
- Acute myocardial infarction
- Wound hematoma
- Prosthetic graft infection
- Acute graft thrombosis
- Late graft occlusion (intimal hyperplasia vs. recurrent atherosclerosis)

Suggested Reading

Leidenfrost J, Geraghty PJ. Peripheral arterial occlusive disease. In: Klingensmith ME, Aziz A, Bharat A, Fox AC, Porembka MR, editors. The Washington manual of surgery. 6th ed. Philadelphia: Lippincott Williams & Wilkins; 2012.

Index

U. Sarpel, *Surgery: An Introductory Guide*,
DOI 10.1007/978-1-4939-0903-2,
© Springer Science+Business Media New York 2014

39838986R00215

Made in the USA
Middletown, DE
26 January 2017